AGEING

AGEING

An Interdisciplinary Approach

Editors
SARJOO PATEL
VEENA GANDOTRA

RAWAT PUBLICATIONS
Jaipur • New Delhi • Bangalore • Hyderabad • Guwahati

ISBN 81-316-0389-X

Published by
Prem Rawat for **Rawat Publications**
Satyam Apts, Sector 3, Jawahar Nagar, Jaipur 302 004 (India)
Phone: 0141 265 1748 / 7006 Fax: 0141 265 1748
E-mail: info@rawatbooks.com
Website: www.rawatbooks.com

New Delhi Office
4858/24, Ansari Road, Daryaganj, New Delhi 110 002
Phone: 011 2326 3290

Also at Bangalore, Hyderabad and Guwahati

Printed at Chaman Enterprises, New Delhi

Dedicated to our beloved parents
with everlasting love and mark of honour,
who made us what we are today.

Contents

	Preface	ix
	Contributors	xiii
1	Senile Miseries and Ways for Resolution *Dimple Saluja*	1
2	Clothing for Elderly People: A Challenge *Madhu Sharan*	9
3	Health Promotion for the Aged: Problems and Solutions in Indian Scenario *Pallavi Mehta and Komal Chauhan*	15
4	Common First Aid Tips for Elderly *Mona Mehta*	27
5	Changes in Clothing Interest of Women during Old Age: A Study *Shivani Verma and Vandana R. Chauhan*	44
6	Ergonomically Designed Toilet Chair: A Remedy to Avoid Accidents Among Old Age People *Nirmal Kaur and Promila Sharma*	56
7	Elderly and Recreation *Babita Shukla*	63

8 Ageing Workforce in the German Labour Market: Review of Intervention Strategies Adopted by Prestigious German Organizations 73
Meeta Agarwal and Veena Gandotra

9 Clothing for Third Age Women 82
Parul Dave and Vandana R. Chauhan

10 Late Middle Age: A Turning Point for Changes in Lifestyle, Diet, Physical Activity and Disease 147
Vanisha S. Nambiar

11 Greying Community of India 157
Varsha Parikh

12 Role and Status of Aged Women: An Analysis of Preferred and Performed Home Role 171
Minaxi Pathak, Ira Bora and Ruplekha Borah

13 Mismatch between Anthropometric Measurements and Dimensions of Toilet Chair: A Cause of Accidents 182
Nirmal Kaur and Promila Sharma

14 Old Age Homes of Baroda: First Hand Encounter 187
Rameshwari Pandya

15 Accidents Among Old Age People While Using Indian Toilet 207
Nirmal Kaur and Promila Sharma

16 Solitude in Old Age 211
Urvashi Pande

17 Age-Defying Foods 223
Vanisha S. Nambiar

18 Time-Use Pattern of Women in the Third Age 231
Maneesha Shukul and Veena Gandotra

19 Safety Measures for Elderly in Old Age Homes 241
Shewanti N. Kashyap

Index 265

Preface

Ageing is a biological process through which every human being passes. It begins at birth and ends with death. It is inevitable, irreversible and progressive increase in the longevity. It cannot be avoided but the rate at which ages vary from country to country and person to person can be checked. It not only depends on one's genes but also on the environmental influences and the lifestyle one follows. The physical abilities slow down but psychological and mental abilities do not deteriorate with age. Thus ageing is a state of mind which does not always keep pace with chronological age. However, for practical purpose, WHO defines people above the age of 60 years as elderly.

India has second largest population of elderly (60+) and it is expected to increase in future too. Demographers have warned that population structure would be more like a pillar than a pyramid as in the past. Average life expectancy in India has increased and by 2011–16 it is projected to be 67 years for males and 69 for females. In next 35 years the number of elderly would be four times more than the present with females outnumbering males.

The transition from adulthood to old age is perceived as a process of loss of physical and mental well-being. The biological and psychological changes are irreversible, which weaken the human ability for survival and adjustment and eventually result in death. Ageing thus brings with it many problems in one's life—both physical as well as psychological. The reduction in vitality increases one's vulnerability to diseases. These changes cannot be prevented but they can be slowed down by proper diet and nutrition. One needs to participate in health education and health promotion activities designed to reduce the risk of diseases. Decreased physical activity and altered metabolism with inadequate regulation of food intake may result in physiological anorexia of ageing (Morley, 1997). The aged are also prone to accidents as their movements becomes restricted with age.

The psychological aspect of ageing also need to be given due consideration. The role and status of aged change as they grow old. The retirement from active work life poses several problems. The loss of productivity—both financial and physical—leads to decline in their status and make them feel worthless and a burden on their children. The physical dependence in later life increases this feeling manifold. The sense of loneliness increases especially if one loses one's spouse. Thus, there is a need to make elderly feel important and useful.

Traditionally, in India, aged enjoyed a place of honour and respect in family and community but in modern times they have lost their place in society. They are replaced by youths in powerful positions leaving them in a weakened and functionless situation. Today, they are viewed as non-productive and dependent lot. Thus, there is a need to look into their problems and provide practical solutions to their physical and psychological needs.

The present book is an attempt to draw attentions to the problems and needs of the ageing population. Learned persons from various disciplines of home sciences have contributed towards this giant issue through their scholarly papers.

To begin with, Dimple Saluja has focused on miseries of senile population and has suggested ways to resolve them. Pallavi Mehta and Komal Chauhan have laid stress on health promotion of the aged focusing on their problems and solutions. Mona Mehta has listed several first aid tips of elderly with focus on what they need to do immediately while facing physiological problems. Madhu Sharan has concentrated on clothing for elderly with their limited mobility and movements. They need such clothes which can be easily worn and removed. Parul Dave and Vandana Chauhan also have put forth some suggestions in their for clothing for women in third age.

Shivani Verma and Vandana Chauhan have studied changing interests of women in their clothing. Nirmal Kaur and Promila Sharma have developed an ergonomically suitable toilet chair for elderly because they discovered that dimensions of toilet chair were not matching with the anthropometric dimensions of elderly. The importance for recreation and the needs of elderly in this respect are highlighted by Babita Shukla in her contribution. Elderly also need their space and have a right to recreational facilities. Meeta Agarwal and Veena Gandotra have reviewed problems of the aged in Germany and have also studied the interventions and strategies developed by various organizations to alleviate the problems of ageing population. Varsha Parikh has focused on the demographic situation and problems of ageing population in India.

Minaxi Pathak, Ira Bora and Ruplekha Borah have analysed the role and status of aged women with focus on domestic chores preferred and performed by women in Assam. Urvashi Pande has highlighted the problem of solitude among the aged, especially those living in old age homes, while Rameshwari Pandya sketches the status of old age homes in Baroda, the facilities they provide and the shortcomings in their provisions. Vanisha Nambiar has discussed about the age defying foods and has provided some dietary guidelines for older people. According to her, late middle age is a turning point in one's life-cycle and if lifestyle modification, dietary changes and adequate physical activities are not initiated, it may lead to the onset of several problems during the old age. Therapeutic lifestyle changes, especially advice of correct diet and physical activity, is the call of the hour. Appropriate advice will not only help in controlling the biochemical indices of the 'moderate' or 'at risk' population, but will also bring down the world wide burden of disease and disability in the aged population. This would inevitably reduce the government's expenditure on health and medicine.

Maneesha Shukul and Veena Gandotra have focused on the time-use patterns of elderly. The changes in use of time are inevitable with elderly after retirement from active work. Shewanti Kashyap has discussed simple modifications in designing the old age homes and carefully selecting the infrastructural facilities to provide a comfortable living to elderly through old age home. Nirmal Kaur and Promila Sharma, in their another paper, have concentrated on the accidents that occurred among the elderly while using Indian toilets. According to them, although changes in body composition are well known, but there is limited knowledge of the changes in anthropometric indices of body composition or the distribution of these changes in the elderly. The authors have also opined that due to the use of Indian toilet by the old age people, the chances of accidents are more because at this stage of life joint problem is very common among them. Thus, to avoid the risk of accidents, the elderly people should have the facility of either the European toilet or if possible the specially made toilet chair.

A book of such a dimension may be of great use to not only elderly, but also the institutions and organizations that are concerned about such people. The editors have thus made an effort to invite experts from various fields of Faculty of Family and Community Sciences (Home Science) to contribute and make this book more meaningful and useful.

Contributors

Babita Shukla, Teaching Assistant, Department of Extension and Communication, Faculty of Family and Community Sciences, Maharaja Sayajirao University of Baroda, Vadodara.

Dimple Saluja, Teaching Assistant, Department of Extension and Communication, Faculty of Family and Community Sciences, Maharaja Sayajirao University of Baroda, Vadodara.

Ira Bora, Department of Family Resource Management, College of Home Science, Assam Agricultural University, Jorhat.

Komal Chauhan, Associate Professor, Department of Foods and Nutrition, a WHO-Collaborating Center for Health Promotion, Faculty of Family and Community Sciences, Maharaja Sayajirao University of Baroda, Vadodara.

Madhu Sharan, Associate Professor, Clothing and Textiles Department, Faculty of Family and Community Sciences, Maharaja Sayajirao University of Baroda, Vadodara.

Maneesha Shukul, Professor, Department of Family and Community Resource Management (Home Management), Faculty of Family and Community Sciences, Maharaja Sayajirao University of Baroda, Vadodara.

Meeta Agarwal, Ex-Training Associate, KVK, Bharsar, G.B. Pant University of Agriculture & Technology, Pantnagar, Uttarakhand.

Minaxi Pathak, Dean, College of Home Science and Head, Department of Family Resource Management, AICRP-FRM Department of Family

Resource Management, College of Home Science, Assam Agricultural University, Jorhat.

Mona Mehta, Teaching Assistant, Department of Family and Community Resource Management (Home Management), Faculty of Family and Community Sciences, Maharaja Sayajirao University of Baroda, Vadodara.

Nirmal Kaur, Assistant Professor, Department of FRM, College of Home Science, G.B. Pant University of Agriculture and Technology, Pantnagar, Uttarakhand.

Pallavi Mehta, Head, Department of Foods and Nutrition, a WHO-Collaborating Center for Health Promotion, Faculty of Family and Community Sciences, Maharaja Sayajirao University of Baroda, Vadodara.

Parul Dave, Director, WSRC, Faculty of Family and Community Sciences, Maharaja Sayajirao University of Baroda, Vadodara.

Promila Sharma, Professor and Head, Department of FRM, College of Home Science, G.B. Pant University of Agriculture and Technology, Pantnagar, Uttarakhand.

Rameshwari Pandya, Associate Professor, Department of Extension and Communication, Faculty of Family and Community Sciences, Maharaja Sayajirao University of Baroda, Vadodara.

Ruplekha Borah, Principal Scientist, AICRP-FRM, Department of Family Resource Management, College of Home Science, Assam Agricultural University, Jorhat.

Shewanti N. Kashyap, Assistant Professor, College of Home Science, Department of Family Resource Management, Rajendra Agriculture University, PUSA, (Samastipur), Bihar.

Shivani Verma, Researcher, Clothing and Textiles Department, Faculty of Family and Community Sciences, Maharaja Sayajirao University of Baroda, Vadodara.

Urvashi Pande, Teaching Assistant, Department of Family and Community Resource Management (Home Management), Faculty of Family and Community Sciences, Maharaja Sayajirao University of Baroda, Vadodara.

Vandana R. Chauhan, Associate Professor, Clothing and Textiles Department, Faculty of Family and Community Sciences, Maharaja Sayajirao University of Baroda Vadodara.

Vanisha S. Nambiar, Assistant Professor, Department of Foods and Nutrition, a WHO-Collaborating Center for Health Promotion, Faculty of Family and Community Sciences, Maharaja Sayajirao University of Baroda, Vadodara.

Varsha Parikh, Teaching Assistant, Department of Extension and Communication, Faculty of Family and Community Sciences, Maharaja Sayajirao University of Baroda, Vadodara.

Veena Gandotra, Ex-Head and Dean, Department of Family and Community Resource Management (Home Management), Faculty of Family and Community Sciences, Maharaja Sayajirao University of Baroda, Vadodara.

1

Senile Miseries and Ways for Resolution

DIMPLE SALUJA

Old age is part of our life cycle. Older persons have always been an integral and important part of the family in Indian society. In the earlier society, the role and the authority of the elders was both supportive and upheld. All ancient and sacred literatures including the Vedas and the epics portray parents almost as God. As a consequence, young people would be differential and respectful towards the elderly. They would abide by the wishes and authority of older persons. Seldom would they think of deviating and protesting against them.

According to Vedas, human life is divided into four ashramas or stages: Brahmacharya (student life), Grihastha (married life), Vanaprastha (life of retirement) and Sanyasa (life of renunciation). The movement from one stage to another was gradual with prescribed specific duties and observances associated with each stage. This minimized inter-stage clash and conflict. When a son would enter into Grihastha ashram, father would usually proceed to Vanaprastha, passing on the responsibilities to the son (Gangrade, 1999).

Yet, another characteristic feature of Indian society is the joint family system. Social traditions sustained and reinforced joint family system as primary social groupings. These joint family groups would among others, function as the upholders of socio-cultural norms, customs and social conventions. A joint family group would be headed by *karta* who would be invariably eldest male, who would oversee assets and liabilities, income and expenditure, adherence to rituals, etc. Taken together, joint family traditions preserved the position of the elderly in the family and society as well. Under this system three generations live together under the some root and all social and economic affairs were controlled and managed within the domain of the household. Hence, the joint family prescribed the way of life and deviation from it was not easy. All this reduces the chances of strain caused by differences within the family.

In the modern times, the social matrix has, however, not remained what it used to be. Commercialization, industrialization and modernization have influenced, modified or even altered many social values and traditions particularly relating to older persons. Even technological changes have adversely affected the older persons. To illustrate, there were earlier a storehouse of anecdotes and stories for grandchildren before TV, video games and comics usurped this role from them. As Soodan (1975) points out that in old age, old people in particular have role less roles.

Apart from this several notable changes are observed in joint family system. Joint family system is being replaced by nuclear family, women accepting paid work outside the household, etc. As such economic and social values have been substantially diluted owing to the loss of relevance of traditional institutions. All this had led to generation gap and has affected the situation of the elderly in society. Gangrade (1999) asserts that Indian society is undergoing transformation under the impact of industrialization, urbanization, commercialization, individualism, etc. Consequently, the traditional values and institutions are under the process of adaptation and have often led to sharpening of inter-generational differences.

Old age is a universal phenomenon and natural biological process of life cycle. For some people it marks the wisdom and experience while for others it can be stage of degeneration characterizing health problems and diseases. Apart from these individual debates, at the macro level, old age poses a serious challenge for policy makers across the globe. Both in developed and developing countries health promotion and primary prevention of disease, better promotion have improved the quality of life and increased the life expectancy. The demographic transition has altered age structure of the population where sizeable proportion in the population is of older persons becoming the norm today.

Concept of Ageing

The human life could be divided into different stages such as childhood, adolescence, adulthood and old age. Traditionally, the term 'elderly' refers to people who have attained certain age chronologically. This caries from country to country and culture to culture. However, for practical purposed, World Health Organization (WHO) calls all persons who are of 60 years and above as the 'elderly' or aged. In the United States of America, the term elderly refers to those who are 65 years and above of age as aged. In India, age limit for the elderly vary from 55 years to 65 years. In the Central government and in mostly state governments, 60 years is the age of superannuation. In private sector and for self-employed people the retirement age is related to health of a person, his disabilities and handicaps associated with advancing age. The decennial Census of India uses the cut off age of 60 years for classifying a person as old.

Ageing is measured in many ways. To a layman, aged is a person who lives longer. Ageing refers to the process of growing older or the effect of age, i.e., the deterioration in physiological capabilities.

Bhatia (1983) defined term 'ageing' from three perspectives: biological, psychological and socio-cultural. Biological ageing refers to bodily changes that occur in the later part of the life of an individual that includes greying of hair, loss of teeth and the diminishing of sight and audibility. Psychological ageing is studied in terms of changes in the nervous system and it consists of general decline in the mental abilities that accompany old age. It also includes the attitude and behaviour of others towards them. Socio-cultural ageing refers to the changes in the individuals, changing circumstances as a member of family, community and society. The changes includes completion of parental roles, retirement from work, reduced income, diseases, disability and need for support. The cultural ageing refers to what behavioural changes mean to the individual and the way internal and external adjustment are made by him.

Mukherji (1972) distinguished between biological, sociological and psychological age. He says biologically a person may be old but if he possesses a youthful mentality, sociologically and psychologically speaking, he should be included in the younger generation. To illustrate this distinction, he cites the example of such leaders as Pandit

Jawaharlal Nehru, Subhas Chandra Bose, Nariman and the like also who in their middle age inspired the youth movement before the Second World War.

According to Tibbittis (1960) ageing may best be defined as the survival of a growing number of people who have completed the traditional adult roles of making a living and child rearing and years following the completion of these tasks, represent and 'extension of life'. It is also said that aged acquire knowledge through experience and so are of much help to the young in a number of ways.

Handler (1960) defines ageing as the deterioration of a nature organism resulting from the dependent, essentially which with the passage of time they became increasingly unable to cope with the stresses of the environment, thereby increasing the probability of death.

Tyagi (1996) defines the aged on the basis of chronological age though, the effect of age on different individuals may vary. For example, in government service a person retires on particular chronological age. A person's physiological, psychological, socio- cultural age is not always linked to chronological age.

So, ageing seems to mean deteriorative biological and psychological changes that occur in genetically matured organism, Indeed these changes are irreversible, weaken the organism's ability for survival and adjustment, and eventually cause the organisms death. Ageing signifies change in roles and status assigned to elders.

Table 1 *Percentage of Population Aged 60 Years and Above (1901–2001)*

Year	*No. of Older Persons (in lakh)*	*Percentage*
1901	12.06	5.06
1911	13.17	5.22
1921	13.48	5.37
1931	14.21	5.09
1941	18.04	5.66
1951	19.61	5.43
1961	24.71	5.63
1971	32.70	5.97
1981	43.98	6.42
1991	55.31	6.55
2001	75.93	7.70

Sources: Ageing in India: Paper No. 2 of 1997, Office of the Registrar General and Census Commissioner of India.

Indian Situation

India too is fast on the path of ageing. On the onset of the 19th century, India had only 5.06 per cent older people (12 million). By 1961, the population of the aged increased to 5.6 per cent (24 million) and by 1981, the aged population almost doubled to 43 million persons. It rose to 6.5 per cent in 1991 and turned to 7.7 per cent in 2001. The proportion of the aged is therefore gradually increasing in the total population.

Table 2 *Percentage of Elderly Persons to Total Population*

Year	*Total Population (In Million)*	*% of Elderly Persons*
2001	70.69	6.90
2006	83.58	7.50
2011	98.47	8.30
2016	118.10	9.30
2021	143.24	10.70
2026	173.00	12.40

Older Persons

India has the second largest population of older (60+) in the world. The number of older persons in the population is expected to increase from 71 million in 2001 to 173 million in 2026. A majority (80%) of the elderly population is a challenge, and there is a large number of 80+ persons in the country

Initiatives for Older Persons during the Tenth Plan

- As contemplated in the National Policy on Older Persons (NPOP), a National Council for Older Persons (reconstituted in 2005) has been set-up to advise and aid the government on policies and programmes for older persons and to provide a feedback to the government on the implementation of NPOP.
- For maintenance and welfare of parents and senior citizens, Citizens Bill, 2007 which has been presented to the parliament, stipulates construction of at least one old age home in each district of the country to accommodate deserving and destitute senior citizens.
- This intended Act will make the process for claiming maintenance simpler, speedier and less expensive. Further, the legislation would also ensure adequate medical facilities to older persons and protection of their life and property.
- The programmes/schemes/incentives for older persons include income tax rebate, higher rates of interest in saving schemes, 30 per cent concessions in all railway travel and 50 per cent

discount on basic fare for all domestic flights in the economy class in Indian Airlines, Jet Airways and other.

- The Ministry of Social Justice and Empowerment implements an integrated programmes for older persons through voluntary organization. Under this schemes, voluntary organization are given 90 per cent grant for running old age homes, day care centres and mobile medical care units. Another schemes for construction of old age homes is being implemented through local self-help groups and voluntary organizations.

The Way Ahead

- The Eleventh Plan proposes to further the right-based approach and also focus on bridging the gap between rural and urban areas.
- A national association for older persons, as per NPOP, will be set-up. Protection of life and property by utilizing the services of panchayats/Senior Citizens Association and other community-based groups and sensitizing and reorienting the law enforcement machinery to the vulnerability and special protection needs of older persons will be taken up in the Eleventh Plan.
- The National Old Age Pension Schemes will now be extended to all below poverty line persons above the age of 60 years. A pension of Rs 200 per month will be provided and states will be requested to add another Rs 200 to this scheme

Policy Recommendations

1. The medical teams consisting of the demographer, the gerontologist, geriatric doctor, the clinical psychologist, the medical/psychiatric/geriatric social worker and geriatric nurses should have to be promoted in the health care of the older persons.
2. Non-governmental organizations (NGOs) and para-professional may have to be actively involve in health care efforts of older persons (both men and women) providing support services for their care, health check-up, nutrition, follow up of medical treatment, etc. Local NGOs could also run day care centre at the gram panchayat, mandal and district levels.
3. Training and research programmes on community-based health care for the elderly in clinical psychology, geriatric, medical and

psychiatric social work, geriatric nursing has to be promoted so as to upgrade the programme.

4. Professional and scientific social work intervention has to be promoted in the prevention, treatment and rehabilitation of psychical, mental and social ill-health.
5. Geriatric health awareness programmes have to be mandatory and inevitable part of social work literacy.
6. Excessive dependence on drugs in geriatric mental health care has to be changed with interpersonal, group and community counselling, community health programmes, social psychiatry and psycho-social work treatment.
7. Geriatric experts may be made readily available at all levels of service.
8. Interpersonal communication, spouse communication, intergenerational communication, etc., should be strengthened so as to promote sustainable standards of geriatric health.
9. The family and the community have to take the responsibility for the elderly as a challenge and more growth opportunities may be made available for improving the quality of their life.
10. Workshops, seminars and conferences on the care of the aged may be organized frequently at various levels as a multi-disciplinary and multi-professional programme.
11. The care programme should include family social work, family therapy, counselling, etc., to prevent family disintegration and to uphold human resource development.
12. Geriatric committees and families to join hands for upgrading the services of the elderly, community day care centre should be scientifically run and professionally equipped. Integrated aged welfare and development projects on the pattern of Integrated Community Development Scheme (ICDS) have to be organized under government sector for each geographical area for care and protection of the aged. The programme should be based on complete involvement of the families and communities including non-governmental organizations (NGOs).
13. Frequent demographic surveys to be conducted to determine the nature and extent of population ageing in various regions and various socio-cultural groups. These surveys are essential to assess the nature and extent of destitution, disability and chronic illness among older persons. Sample surveys are also required to assess morbidity patterns and healthy/disease-free life expectancy.

14. Physical beautification, environmental sanitation, personal hygiene, horticultural therapy, music therapy and occupational therapy have to be promoted and strengthened.
15. Strengthening of family betterment committees.
16. Including detailed care programmes of elderly in family social work courses.
17. Psychosocial and economic betterment and empowerment of women and families are essential to cater to care of the older persons.
18. Journalist and mass media should cover care programmes of older persons in totality.

Conclusion

When all is said and done, our attitude towards the old determines our actions/or them. The old are to be cared for cherished and comforted because that are 'valuable human resource' that have done with voyaging and are laden with the wealth of experience. Give them respect which they richly deserve. By providing the onerous services to the aged, the individual, the family, the society and the state ensures that the years of retirement as those who have worked and toiled hard in its service shall be free from anxiety, want and boredom.

References

Bhatia, H.S. (1983), *Ageing and Society: A Sociological Study of Retired Public Servants*. New Delhi, Arya Book Centre.

Eleventh Five-Year Plan, (2007–2012), Planning Commission, Government of India, Volume III, Agriculture, Rural Development, Industry Services and Physical Infrastructure.

Gangrade, K.D. (1999), "Emerging Conception of Ageing is India: A Socio-cultural Perspective". In Bali, Arun P. (ed.), *Understanding Graying People of India*, New Delhi, Inter India Publications.

Handler, P. (1960), "Radiation and Ageing In Stock". N.W. (ed.), *Ageing Washington* D.C. American Association for the Advancement of Science.

Nasreen, Asiya, (2009). *Urban Eldeuly Coping Strategies and Societal Responses*. Concept Publications, New Delhi, p. 13, 14, 16, 17, 21.

Soodan. K.S. (1975), *Ageing in India*, Calcutta, Minerva.

Thara Bhai. L. (2002), *Integrated Approach to Old Age Care: Problems and Prospects*, Decent Books, New Delhi, pp. 114–116.

Tibittis, C. (1960), *Handbook of Social Gerontology*, Chicago, University of Chicago Press.

2

Clothing for Elderly People

A Challenge

MADHU SHARAN

Clothing has been identified as one of the basic needs of the human being other than food and shelter. Human being uses clothes from cradle to grave, i.e., throughout the life but requirement in details of clothing changes with age. Peoples of different age have different clothing requirement. Other factors like environment, job profile, status, society also dictates the requirement of the clothes. Clothing plays a double role in social interactions, i.e., forming the first impression of the person and affecting the action of the wearer. Today market is flooded with clothes of many varieties at different prices catering to the needs of the people. Clothing needs can be broadly classified as (i) general needs, and (ii) special needs.

General Needs

These are common to nearly all garments. It includes: (a) *Protection*—Clothing provide protection against weather, plants, animals and insects. This is important for infants and elderly who are most vulnerable, immobile and least able to care for themselves. (b) *Safety*—Functionally well designed clothes eliminates many health hazards like injuries due to fire, road accidents and provide comfort, efficiency and safety. (c) *Decoration*—Clothes if properly selected enhances the personality of the wearer. It is used to hide or highlight certain features of the wearer. It serves only visual purpose. (d) *Identification*—Many a time clothes provide identification to an individual, e.g., uniforms. It also conveys the individual's recognition to certain group and culture. Prevailing social norms and attitudes are often reflected in the clothing.

Special Needs

Some people require special considerations in clothing. They are identified as persons with special needs who require and deserve professional and consumer attention. They too, want to feel attractive and gain social acceptance. Among those requiring special consideration are those in certain occupations, children, pregnant women, the handicapped and the elderly. For each of these groups, good functional designed clothes become very important.

Clothing for the elderly needs to be given attention as they (elderly) also hold a significant position in the family. Even though they form a relatively small market, it is a significant one. The percentage of elderly people in population around the world is rising as life expectancies has increased due to advances in the medical sciences. It has brought many new problems, some of which has implications on clothing also. The fairly low fixed incomes, fixed preferences and increasing immobility which leads to less wear and tear of clothes of many of the old age people results in minimum consumption of clothes. Mental and psychological capabilities and interests often continues while physical capabilities decline. Major problems arise due to physical change in the body like stooped shoulders, joint and finger stiffness, upper arm and neck flabbiness, thickened waists which needs to be considered while designing so as to accommodate these physical changes comfortably and attractively. With the age there is less body-temperature control and increased susceptibility to hypothermia (reduced body temperature control). Researches has shown that many elderly people perceive clothing as a useful tool to increase their control over body temperature. The human figure usually changes in size and proportion as they grow older. There is often an increase in weight and a decrease in height. Weight gradually increases from the middle years to about the age of seventy when it begins to decrease. With a decrease in physical strength and energy, thought must be given to designing clothes which are easy to put on and take off, and easy to care for. With changing bodily characteristics, it is necessary to solve the problems of fitting the mature figure and of designs and colours which are becoming to this age group; and with decreasing earning power and hence income, one must consider the original cost and the maintenance cost of the clothes for them. Amongst the all the most difficult physical changes to adjust are those related to general health, i.e., the loss of energy and vigour. The elderly also need affection and recognition of their personal dignity. They do not want to be singled out and pitied. Clothing is such an important part of a senior's overall mental health. That is because attitude makes all the difference in their lives. And looking good is an important part of feeling good.

Clothing expectations for various age categories are seldom enforced as rigidly as they are for sex roles. Incongruities between age and dress are obvious, not only because they highlight the individual's physical disparities, but because they are essentially in violation of the normative expectation. Men in their seventies are expected to pay greater attention to their physical comforts in clothes and their overall appearance is anticipated to be somewhat relaxed and subdued. Older people want to make a good impression and wish to give a dignified appearance through more formal clothing.

Problems Related to Clothing during Old Age

The body not only gains in weight after the middle years but the distribution of weight also shifts. The body fat tends to move slowly downward—"the bust or chest becomes relatively smaller and the abdomen and hips larger". Often the waistline disappears entirely and the body becomes almost pear shaped. The shoulders become rounded and there is a roll of fat at the base of neck in back. Another problem is the loss of fat in the upper arms. This causes an unattractive sagging of the flesh and an increase in wrinkles at some part of the body. Many older people are afflicted with arthritis and other diseases of the joints and muscles which leads to lesser pliability and flexibility. There is increased susceptibility to both heat and cold. The ageing body loses its resiliency and power of adaptation and regulation. The elderly tend to move less and more slowly and thus do not have the warmth generated by the movement. Also there is a loss of a layer of subcutaneous fat which serves as a layer of insulation during younger age. Thus older people are more sensitive to both cold and heat. There is declining amount of enjoyment in shopping for clothing because of reasons not being able to find clothing they liked and which fit, becoming tired easily. Older people are more conservative in their clothing than younger people. They choose more subdued colours and more classic styles as they feel these are the only garments available in sizes which fit them, expect conservative clothes last longer.

Solutions

The half-size dresses which have a larger waistline are a partial answer to the need, i.e., change in waistline. Extra fullness is needed in the back, and the length between the neckline and the waistline usually needs to be increased if the garment is to be hanged correctly. Dress should be designed with a sleeve which covers the arm to a point below the elbow. With a decrease in energy and vigour and stiffening of the muscles, even those in relatively good health need garments which do not require extensive stretching and reaching to put on or to fasten and unfasten. Dresses which open in the front are satisfactory in this respect. Larger armholes such as those for raglan sleeves are also easier to put on. Clothing which are warmer in winter and cooler in summer and can be put on or removed with ease should be used. Dress designs which emphasize the waistline should not be used. Arrangements should be made so that the sales personnel bring garments to them rather than having racks of dresses which they have to look through themselves. Provision of better lightings and wider racks should be there. They should be provided with better fitting clothes.

To cope up with their falling health, elderly people are advised to do some physical exercise. To make them comfortable during exercise, selection of appropriate clothing plays an important role. All exercise clothing should be loose-fitting to permit freedom of movement, and should make one feel comfortable and self-assured. They should wear lighter clothes than temperatures might indicate. Exercise generates great amounts of body heat. Light-coloured clothing that reflects the sun's rays is cooler in the summer, and dark clothes are warmer in the winter. When the weather is very cold, it is better to wear several layers of light clothing than one or two heavy layers. The extra layers help trap heat, and it is easier to shed one of them if it become too warm. In cold weather, and in hot sunny weather, it is a good to wear something on head. Wool caps are recommended for winter wear, and some form of hat that provides shade is good for summer. Rubberized or plastic clothing should never be used. Such garments interfere with the evaporation of perspiration and can cause body temperature to rise to dangerous levels.

Some other informal clothes recommended for elderly are:

1. A wrap-around garment with velcro closures.
2. A reversible front-to-back gown or caftan.
3. A full-length garment with elbow-length or long sleeves.
4. A stylish pajama with velcro for both men and women.
5. Shirt with false buttons down the front that is secured with velcro.
6. Sportswear fashions such as stylish tracksuits for exercise.
7. Tops that fasten at the shoulders.

Functionality is also important in their clothes. Use of large buttons, velcro snaps in place of smaller buttons, replacement of traditional zippers that are easier for arthritic hands to manoeuver are desirable features in their clothing.

A pleasant appearance gives a lift to almost anyone and elderly are no exceptions. A person who is dressed and groomed neatly and attractively is less likely to be filled with self-pity, and he is more sociable. The older person who feels that his appearance is acceptable is more likely to participate socially. The older individual is still interested in clothing and is motivated to look attractive to others. Individuals use clothing to foster self-esteem and to assist in social encounter. Daily choice of personal attire remains one way by which elderly individuals in institutions may express feelings about self and attitudes towards others. The majority of elderly men wants clothing that are comfortable, up-to-date, and like that of their friends. Clothing is considered to enhance self-confidence and to assist in impressive management. Men who were less active in the leisure role show greater interest in the psychological and social components of clothing. With people living longer, there is a need for clothing for the frail and those with special needs. Many seniors have mobility and health issues brought on by surgeries, illnesses or other conditions like arthritis. When you are shopping or designing for seniors, choosing both functional and stylish fashions is important to their health and well-being.

Select References

Davis, Marian L. (1972) *Visual Design in Dress*. Prentice-Hall, Inc., Englewood Cliffs, New Jersey, pp. 10–15.

Kathryn, M. and M. Janine. (1989) *Fashion Design: Process, Innovation and Practice*. Blackwell Science, Oxford, pp. 29–41.

Marilyn, J.H. (1968) *The Second Skin: An Interdisciplinary Study of Clothing*. Houghton Mifflin Company, Boston, pp. 2–12.

Mary, S.R. (1965) *Clothing: A Study in Human Behaviour*. Holt, Rinehart and Winston, Inc., New York, pp. 306–323.

Simpson, M.M. and M.A. Littrell. (1984) "Attitudes toward Clothing of Elderly Men". *Journal of Applied Gerontology*, Vol. 3, No. 2, pp. 171–173.

3

Health Promotion for the Aged

Problems and Solutions in Indian Scenario

PALLAVI MEHTA AND KOMAL CHAUHAN

Ageing is continues biological process that begins at birth and ends with death. Its inevitable, irreversible and progressive increase in longevity all over the world has created interest in geriatric science. Poor control over birth rates and rapid decline in death rates have resulted increase in numbers of both the aged and children resulting in a larger number of dependents.

Demographers have already warned that the population structure is transiting from pyramid to pillar. By 2025, 10 per cent of the total population in India will be of the age 60 years and above. The 'grey' population is getting more mature. About 10 per cent of the population over 60 years of age is in the age bracket of 80 years and this will rise to 25 per cent by the year 2050. Expectation of life at birth for males and females has increased more in recent years. In India, it is projected to be 67 years by 2011–16 for males and 69 years for females. Projections beyond 2016 made by United Nations (1990) as per the sex and age distribution of population, has indicated that 21 per cent of the Indian population will be 60+ by 2050 which was 6.8 per cent in 1991 (Bose and Shankerdass, 2001). In the next 35 years their number will be four times as high as today with females outnumbering males. Data available on health and nutritional status of elderly women with different living arrangements is scarce.

The transition from adulthood to old age is often perceived as a process of loss of physical and psychological health status. Health needs and problems of the elderly are many and varied. With advancing age there is a reduced vitality and increased vulnerability to common diseases both acute and chronic. The social changes that accompany urbanization are likely to increase nutritional risk for this age group.

Despite lower energy intakes with age, elderly have higher requirements for several micronutrients, making them vulnerable to deficiencies that further aggravate chronic conditions.

After fifty years of age there are many metabolic and physiological changes, which show an impact on the nutritional needs of an individual. The metabolic rate slows and can decline as much as thirty per cent over a lifetime. This results in decreased caloric needs, which can be complicated by changes in an older person's ability to balance food intake and energy needs. Even with a decreased caloric need, many older people have difficulty getting sufficient calories, which can eventually lead to chronic fatigue, depression, and a weakened immune system. Decreased physical activity and altered metabolism with ageing fail to adequately regulate food intake and results in physiological anorexia of ageing (Morley, 1997).

While there are many physical and clinical factors that can contribute to undernutrition in the elderly, there are as many equally important social and economic factors, which can further complicate the nutritional well-being of an older individual. Contributing factors include loneliness, lack of cooking skills, depression, economic concerns, weakness and fatigue, and, in too many cases, an unwarranted fear of many high quality, nutrient dense, affordable foods. All these factors can contribute to the fact that a significant number of older men and women consume less food than required to meet energy and nutrient requirements, and are at moderate to high nutritional deficiency risk.

Arthritis makes it difficult for the elderly living alone to shop for and prepare food. A decreased ability to taste and smell can also affect the enjoyment of food. For the elderly, poor dentition, loss of teeth and poorly fitted dentures can cause chewing problems and mouth sores, making eating process difficult.

Those living alone and who face financial difficulties tend to skip on food, and may cook only one dish a day to be eaten over breakfast, lunch and dinner. Many elderly men neglect their nutrition because they lack the cooking skills and knowledge about nutrition (especially after the death of the spouse), suffers from problems such as loneliness and depression, or weakness and fatigue. Others consume too much deep-fried, oily food instead of more nutrient-dense foods like fruit, vegetables and whole grains (Health Promotion Board, 2005).

Another possible factor is lack of knowledge. In many societies, men, particularly may not have knowledge of food preparation and are therefore compromising a lot on proper dietary intake, ultimately they are most at risk.

In a study reported earlier by Mehta et al. (1997), diminished food intake, depression and negative thoughts were also seen more in the institutionalized elderly as compared to the elderly living with family.

Living arrangements are a key dimension of quality of life and well-being in old age. Availability of family care, as well as social and economic support, is in part a function of which you live with.

Thus, the problems causing malnutrition among the elderly include: physical incapacity to obtain and/or prepare food, cognitive problems, medical conditions requiring dietary changes, poor dental health (badly fitting dentures can make it painful and difficult to eat), trouble in chewing and/or swallowing, loss of the sense of smell or taste makes food unattractive, an unrecognized infection in the urinary tract can make people feel too ill to want to eat. Bowel problems such as severe constipation cause pain and make people unwilling to eat. Due to high consumption of alcohol, social isolation and/or depression, older people may fail to recognize when they are thirsty and even certain problems with their mobility can stop them getting themselves a drink leading to dehydration at a longer period of time. Dehydration is a common risk in older people and a dry mouth makes food hard to chew or swallow. Therefore ideally water or a drink should always be served with their meals. Digesting solid food takes a lot of energy, so the act of eating a meal can be tiring to a frail person. Recent life events such as bereavement, or an unwanted move to a new place to live, or loss of contact with friends can diminish appetite due to grief. Many people lose interest in food when they no longer have someone with whom to share their meals. Uses of multiple medications, advanced age (80+) and malnutrition have serious negative health consequences for seniors. The progressive effects of malnutrition in elderly people include: loss of muscle mass, weakness and fatigue, impaired immune response, poor wound healing, impaired organ function, infection, sepsis and without nutritional intervention, death.

Physiological Changes which Affect Nutrient and Food Intake during Ageing Process

- Reduced metabolism—Low BMR, lack of physical activity, lack of appetite, reduced food intake, multiple nutritional deficiency.
- Loss of teeth and difficulty in mastication, altered food intake, liquid, soft mashy diet, low nutrient intake, avoidance of vegetables and fruits.
- Taste buds atrophy, alteration of threshold of certain tastes leading to altered food preferences, more sweet and salty foods, difficult control of diabetes and hypertension, which are common in old age.
- Reduction of gastric volume, altered meal pattern and gastric dysfunction, delayed emptying rate of stomach, altered food intake and avoidance of many foods.
- Atrophy of gastro-intestinal tract musculature, reduced intestinal motility, GIT disorders and reduced food intake.

Given below in Table 1 are the contributory factors responsible for nutritional problems in elderly people.

Table 1 *Potential Contributors to Nutritional Problems in Elderly People*

Physical Factors	*Social and Psychological Factors*
Reduced total energy needs	Depression
Declining absorptive and metabolic capacities	Loneliness
Chronic diseases	Social isolation
Anorexia	Bereavement
Changes in taste/odour perception	Loss of interest in food or cooking
Poor dentition	Mental disorders
Reduced salivary flow	Food faddism
Dysphasia	Socioeconomic factors
Lack of exercise	Inadequate cooking or storage facilities
Physical disability (restricting the capacity to purchase, cook, or eat a varied diet)	Poor nutrition knowledge
Drug-nutrient interactions	Lack of transportation
Side effect of drugs (anorexia, nausea, altered taste)	Shopping difficulties
Restrictive diets and alcoholism	Cooking practices (resulting in nutrient losses)
Inadequate cooking skills (men)	

Source: Horwath, (1989).

Strategies to Combat Health Problems

The scenario can change if the elderly who are a neglected class of population are offered special dietetic care in addition to medical facilities. There are foods and formulas available commercially for infants and children. However there are no special foods available for the geriatric group of people. Many elderly have difficulty in getting and making home made food because of problems with food related activities ranging from purchasing to eating, lack of resources, absence of spouse and physical health problems. Well balanced formulations in the form of ready to use mixes or easy to make and digest foods can serve as the best convenience foods for this population. In order to suite the target group and for good acceptability, these foods should have certain characteristics like low viscosity, nutrient density, good fibre content and high digestibility. Care should also be taken to design foods which are low cost, low in fat and flatulence factor, easy to chew and swallow and yet acceptable to the ageing palate. Feeding oneself with such nutritious food will add to self-confidence, feeling of security and improvement in the health status leading to high self-esteem and ability to carry out various activities.

All the above observations therefore indicate a need to identify the nutritional problems by designing suitable modifications.

At all ages over 65 years, there are more women than men in our society. Despite their lower mortality rates, older women have greater morbidity, including more limitations in self-care. Financially also, women are dependent on others therefore they neglect on their health problems. Since on average women live longer than men, the health problems of older adults, in reality, are often those of older women. Nutritional problems are especially prevalent in the elderly women and require appropriate counselling in long-term management. Age-related declines in gastrointestinal and bone marrow functional reserve have been found to occur in elderly. The elderly have decreased physical activity, changed and poor dietary pattern. They also have increased frequency of inflammatory processes. These factors prove to develop anaemia (Olivares et al., 1999).

The present authors have attempted to conduct some intervention trials through several studies to tackle the problems of the elderly. Findings of the studies are summarized below.

Mehta et al. (1997) studied prevalence of disease profile among elderly men and women in different income groups. They found that prevalence of oral cavity and gastrointestinal problems were higher followed by central nervous system and locomotors problems irrespective to income groups.

The work on local elderly population in Vadodara city by the same team included a study on 166 men (mean age 62 years) and 70 (mean age 58 years) women aged 45 years and above. They showed similar occurrence of problems among elderly men and women. Locomotor problems were more prevalent in elderly women especially selected for the study (Shringarpure, 2004).

In an interesting study on thirst, fluid and urine excretion pattern among 50 older adults and 50 local elderly subjects, investigators reported that prevalence of viral fever, infections and diarrhoeal episodes were found higher in elderly as compared to younger women and thus showing that elderly people are more at risk of dehydration (Ray et al., 2006).

The team have shown similar occurrence of problems among elderly men and women (Mehta et al., 1997).

Another study on food preferences and taste sensitivity of local elderly women residing in Vadodara city revealed that there was a change in preference for certain class of foods and a decline in taste sensitivity with the advancement of age (Mehta et al., 2007). The food items developed were more preferred by the elderly women than the younger panel members. Figure 1 shows the acceptability of various foods by the subjects belonging to two age groups.

Figure 1 *Comparison between the Two Age Group Subjects for the Acceptability of the Various Food Items*

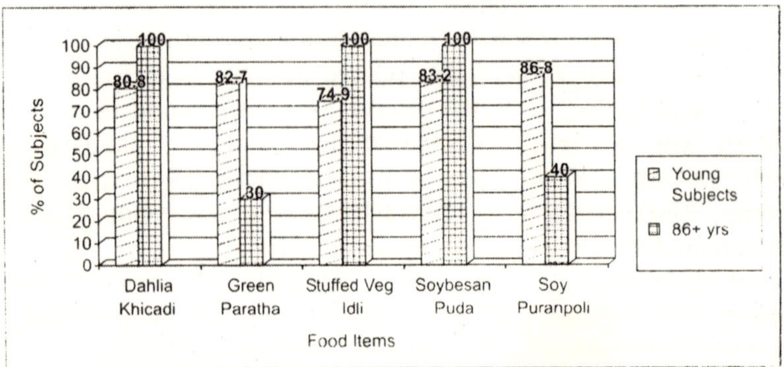

Intervention Measures

Intervention studies that were carried out with supplementation of nutrient, foods or nutrition health education showed beneficial effect on the overall health of the elderly, especially on elderly anaemic subjects.

Since prevalence of anaemia in older individuals is about 50 per cent in developing countries and 12 per cent in developed countries (WHO, 2000) and is a risk factor for subsequent decline in physical performance, cognitive functions and increased morbidities in older persons, one of the suggested strategies for prevention and treatment of anaemia are supplementation with iron.

A study conducted on elderly anaemic women showed beneficial effect of iron folic acid tablet supplementation on physical performance and cognitive function test of the subjects (Mehta et al., 2005). Three hundred elderly (60 years and above) women as subjects were screened for anaemia through haemoglobin estimation from free-living population living under major five zones of Vadodara. Further from the anaemic group, 60 subjects were selected and divided in control and experimental group respectively. Iron folic acid tablet supplementation and nutrition health education (NHE) for a period of six weeks was given to experimental group elderly women.

Salient findings of the study were:

- Anaemic elderly subjects face more daily activity problems as compared to the non-anaemic ones.
- Iron folic acid supplementation for six weeks was found effective method for combating iron deficiency anaemia reflecting on physical performance and cognitive function tests.
- Use of pictured NHE booklet along with verbal counselling seemed to be effective in bringing awareness regarding the risk factors as well as preventive aspects of iron deficiency anaemia.

In another study the problems of food related activity among elderly women were assessed in elderly women subjects, which included problems faced during purchasing, storing, cooking and eating. Results showed that elderly women living alone bared maximum difficulties in various food related activities and had poor health and nutritional status followed by elderly women living with spouse and with children. Thus it was felt that there was a need to develop nutritious and quick cooking food items which would help to improve the health and nutritional status of the elderly. Further soy as functional food was selected and few food items like soy sambhar, soy paratha, soy dhokli and soy usal were developed and evaluated. This food items contained 12–15 gms of protein with a sensory scores of 7.0 and above on 9.0 point hedonic rating scale (Chauhan, 2007).

An earlier study by Anuradha Limaye (1999) on institutionalized elderly showed poor nutrition and health profile. A study was undertaken on institutionalized elderly using soy-based products and its impact on health and nutritional status of subjects was assessed. Soy food items stated above were given daily for three months showed improvement in the nutrients intake, haemoglobin levels, lipid profile, minor illnesses and general well-being of the institutionalized elderly (Chauhan, 2007). Table 2 shows the percentage of institutionalized elderly men and women reporting minor illnesses before and after three months of intervention with soy supplementation.

Table 2 *Percentage of Institutionalized Elderly Men and Women Reporting Minor Illnesses Before and After Three Months of Intervention with Soy Supplementation*

Minor Illnesses	*Before Intervention*			*After Intervention*		
	Males (n=14)	*Females (n=6)*	*Total (n=20)*	*Males (n=14)*	*Females (n=6)*	*Total (n=20)*
Cold and cough	29(4)	33(2)	30(6)	—	—	—
Fever	14(2)	33(2)	20(4)	—	—	—
Infections	36(5)	50(3)	40(8)	21(3)	33(2)	25(5)
Vomiting and diarrhoea	43(6)	33(2)	40(8)	29(4)	17(1)	25(5)
Constipation	64(9)	67(4)	65(13)	50(7)	33(2)	45(9)
Indigestion	50(7)	50(3)	50(10)	29(4)	17(1)	25(5)
Body aches	71(10)	67(4)	70(14)	43(6)	33(2)	40(8)
Pain in joints	57(8)	33(2)	50(10)	36(5)	—	25(5)
Dizziness	29(4)	17(1)	25(5)	—	—	—

Figures in the parentheses denote number of subjects.

Table 2 showed that soy supplementation was found to be hypo-cholesterolemic with improvement in HDL-cholesterol and reduction in LDL-cholesterol levels, which proved beneficial effect on health of the subjects. Table 3 depicts the mean values for the lipid profile of institutionalized elderly subjects before and after three months of intervention with soy supplementation.

Table 3 *Mean Values of the Lipid Profile of Institutionalized Elderly before and after three Months of Intervention with Soy Supplementation (n=18)*

Parameters	*Initial Mean ± SD*	*3 Months Intervention Mean ± SD*	*'t' Value*
Total Cholesterol (mg/dl)	173.05 ± 23.68	170.9 ± 17.3	0.78
Triglycerrides (mg/dl)	125.8 ± 11.69	127.7 ± 10.2	-1.72
HDL (mg/dl)	37.83 ± 2.79	41.83 ± 2.20	-6.73*
VLDL (mg/dl)	25.1 ± 2.3	24.8 ± 2.4	0.51
LDL (mg/dl)	108.4 ± 24.1	104.66 ± 1.46	1.70*
TC/HDL	4.54 ± 0.6	4.12 ± 0.4	4.41*
LDL/HDL	2.83 ± 0.63	2.52 ± 0.44	3.42*

* Significant at $p < 0.05$.

Geriatric research team of the department also attempted to study KAP (Knowledge, Attitude and Practice) of the caregivers of the elderly. This study data on evaluation of NHE intervention in selected elderly caregivers showed that many of the caregivers had knowledge, retention and followed the same practice regarding almost all aspects of elderly overall health care (Panchal et al., 2005).

Mental health of the elderly also has influence in the overall health of the elderly. Depression is one of the most common mental disorders found which is referred as the 'common cold' among mental illnesses. Depression poses a major public health challenge in the coming years. Literature has shown higher rates of depression among older adults especially women. According to a study carried out by WSRC, (2005) on mental health and ageing, the causes of higher rates of depression in women are numerous and are often a mix of biological (hormonal fluctuations throughout life span, malnutrition and greater burden of reproductive health related problems) and psychological and cultural factors (poverty, powerlessness, unequal work distribution and workload, low self-esteem, low status in the family, experience of violence, abuse and stressful life). Depression in old women increases due to process of ageing, poor health, undernutrition, loss of spouse and other significant relations, insecurity, etc. In their study they found that 42 per cent women had moderate depression. This makes the elderly more vulnerable, ultimately affecting their health and nutritional status. In the same interdisciplinary study Mehta et al. (2002) assessed the nutritional status of depressed elderly women. Findings showed the positive improvement in the nutrients intake with iron folic acid supplementation for a period of two months on the moderately depressed elderly women. Table 4 shows the impact of intervention on the nutrients intake of the subjects.

Table 4 *Mean Nutrient Intake of Depressed Elderly Women before and after Iron Folic Acid Supplementation (n=30)*

Nutrients	*Mean*		*P-value*
	Pre-intervention	*Post-intervention*	
Energy (Kcal)	1,269	1,701	*0.00
Protein (gm)	28.03	62.93	*0.00
Iron (mg)	18.19	36.54	*0.00
Folic acid (mg)	59.29	148.40	*0.00
Calcium (mg)	236	611	*0.00
Vitamin C (mg)	20.32	45.31	*0.00

Significant *p<0.05.

In a study by Mehta et al. (2008) on 15 moderately depressed elderly women Brahmi was given (750 mg of *bacopa monira*/day) for a period of six weeks. Results on mental health status showed a significant improvement (p≤0.05) in the depression level using Beck's Depression Inventory scale (BDI). A shift of 86.6 per cent subjects (*n*=15) into mild and 13.3 per cent into normal category of mini mental state examination test scores was noticed. A significant increase was also found in the mean nutrient intake like energy, protein, choline, tryptophan and methionine (p≤0.05).

Patil (2007) supplemented herb Ashwagandha for six weeks to 15 moderately depressed elderly women and also found similar improvements in the mental health status along with significant improvement in mean haemoglobin levels (10.4 gm% improved to 10.9 gm%, p≤0.05) and mean weight (44.65 gm% to 45.6 gm%, p≤0.05).

Thus, intervention had profound effect in improving the health and nutritional status of the elderly. Health promotion also focused at educating community at large.

Considering this, there are some important issues before the teaching colleges:

- To include in teaching/training curriculum, the essentials of appropriate clinical approach to the health care of the elderly.
- To teach students to identify and be aware of unusual/a typical manifestations of disease due to multiple illness and multiple drug therapy in the elderly.
- To develop special skills to interview techniques in case of the elderly and special approach to planning management.
- Geriatric health is a specialized discipline and development of integrated teaching is required.
- Geriatric care team concept has to be developed and inculcated.

— Preventive geriatrics mainly deals with modifying lifestyles and environmental factors in order to prevent ill-health (primary prevention).

— Early reporting of illness leading to prompt management (secondary prevention).

— Early initiation of rehabilitation (tertiary prevention).

This can enable the elderly to regain and maintain the possible level of activities of daily living.

References

Bose, A and Shankerdass, S. (2001), *Growing Old in India*, Tata McGraw Publication, New Delhi.

Chauhan, Komal. (2007) Health Promotion for the Aged Through Intervention with Suitable Foods and Nutrient Supplementation. Unpublished Ph.D. Dissertation, Dept. of Foods and Nutrition, Faculty of Family and Community Sciences, M.S. University of Baroda, Vadodara.

Health Promotion Board. (2001) Health A-Z Online, Nutrition for the Elderly, Singapore.

Horwath, C.C. (1989) "Socio-economic Status and Dietary Habits in the Elderly: Results from a Large Random Survey". *Journal of Nutrition and Dietetics*, Volume 2, pp. 173–83.

Limaye, A. (1999) A Study on Diet, Nutrition and Health Profile of Institutionalised and Non-institutionalised Elderly of Baroda city (60 years and above). Unpublished Master's Dissertation, Dept. of Foods and Nutrition,

Faculty of Family and Community Sciences, M.S. University of Baroda, Vadodara.

Mehta, Pallavi, Komal Chauhan and Chayanika Devi. (2007) "Study on Food Preferences and Taste Sensitivity of Local Elderly Women Residing in Baroda City and Evaluation of Selected Food Items for Geriatric Group". *Ind J Geront*, Vol. 21, No. 1, pp. 20–29.

Mehta, Pallavi, Komal Chauhan and Swati Parnami. (2005) "A Study on Nutrition, Diet and Disease Profile of the Elderly Anemic Women (aged 60 yrs and above) with and without Intervention with Iron Folic Acid Supplementation". *Ind J Geront*, Vol. 19, No. 1, pp. 40–49.

Mehta, Pallavi, Monisha Vyas and Mini Sheth. (1997) Reaching the Unreached, Part I, Monograph published by Dept. of Foods and Nutrition, Faculty of Family and Community Sciences, M.S. University of Baroda, Vadodara.

Mehta, Pallavi, Tejal Vasavda, Arpita Shah and Komal Chauhan. (2008) "Brahmi: An Alternative Therapy for Depression in Elderly Women" in by Parul Dave and Pallavi Mehta (eds.), *Mental Health and Ageing Women: Important Correlates*. Kalpaz Publications, Delhi, pp. 474–82.

Morley, J.E. (1997) "Foods for Thought". *Am J of Clin Nutr*, Vol. 66, No. 4, pp. 760–63.

Olivares, M. Herstramph, E., Capuriro, H.T. and Wenger, D. (1999), "Prevalence of Anemia in Elderly Subjects Living at Home: Role of Micronutrient Deficiency and Inflammation". *European Journal of Clinical Nutrition*, pp. 54, 834–839.

Panchal, Nirali, Komal Chauhan and Pallavi Mehta. (2005) "Study on Knowledge and Practices of Caregivers of the Elderly (> 75 yrs) and Impact of Nutrition Health Education on Elderly Health". *Ind J Geront*, Vol. 19, No. 4, pp. 152–158.

Patil, Gauri. (2007) A Study on Nutrition and Health Profile of Depressed Elderly Women of Baroda City: Impact of Herbal Intervention with Ashwagandha on Mental Health of Elderly Women. Unpublished M.Sc Dissertation, Dept. of Foods and Nutrition, Faculty of Family and Community Sciences, M.S. University of Baroda, Vadodara.

Ray, Sheetal, Pallavi Mehta and Komal Chauhan. (2006) "A Study on Thirst, Fluid Intake and Urine Excretion Pattern of Older Adult and Elderly Females residing in Vadodara City". *J Ind Diet Assoc*, Vol. 31, Nos. 1 and 2, pp. 31–36.

Shringarpure, Bhagyashree. (2004) Role of Antioxidants during Ageing. Unpublished Ph.D. Dissertation, Dept. of Foods and Nutrition, Faculty of Family and Community Sciences, M.S. University of Baroda, Vadodara.

WSRC. (2005) Project Report on Mental Health and Ageing: Focus on Women with Depression. Women's Studies Research Centre, M.S. University of Baroda, Vadodara.

4

Common First Aid Tips for Elderly

MONA MEHTA

Accidents/disasters are common among all groups whether it be doctors, nurses, ambulance crews, police, or any businessman. The experts from the various health institutions precisely know what to do and in what order to do to solve basic accidental problems. But probably the elderly in the home are unaware of the basic common first aid treatment that should be given in case of accidents like breathing problems, acute asthma, severe strokes, burning, fainting, head injuries and drowning. The present paper attempts to focus on the various common tips to be followed while facing such life accidents. It aims to give knowledge to the elderly in handling an emergency on the spot in case it happens with any one of their own family members. It also helps them to deal with some common disasters sensibly rather than being caught unaware.

Breathing

Breathing is the process by which air is drawn into the chest through the nose and mouth and is then blown out again through the same passages. Whilst in the chest, or more precisely the lungs, the air gives up some of its oxygen (about one-fifth) and this is taken into the blood circulation; in return the blood gives up the same amount of its waste product, carbon dioxide. This process is a continuous one from the time of birth to the time of death, and is often visible and obvious. If breathing stops, then within three or four time minutes the heart will fail. The chest wall will not be moving up and down.

The stomach wall will not be moving in and out. Therefore, one must start artificial breathing or artificial respiration immediately. The kiss of life (mouth-to-mouth respiration) is the simplest and recommended method, and artificial respiration is only used in special cases. The aim of the kiss of life is to do the work of breathing when the casualty cannot do it himself.

The Kiss of Life

1. If it is possible to get someone else to call an ambulance, this is the first thing you arrange, but every second counts and you do not have time to do this yourself. If there is no one to do this for you, it must wait until the patient has received first aid.
2. Turn the casualty, when possible, so that he is lying on his back.
3. Loosen clothing round casualty's neck, chest and waist.
4. Clean casualty's mouth and nose, and remove any dentures, vomit, food or saliva, using a tissue or handkerchief over your fingers.
5. Place one of your hand under the neck and the other on the forehead so that the casualty's head is titled backwards.
6. Using the hand from under the neck, lift the chin upwards. This simple procedure often clears the airway, when the casualty will take a breath and start to breathe on his own. But it is important to keep the breath and start to breathe on his own. But it is important to keep the head in this position for the clear airway to be maintained until consciousness returns.
7. However, if breathing does not start, pinch the casualty's nostrils together, take in a breath yourself, cover casualty's mouth completely and firmly with yours, and breathe into his lungs.
8. From the corner of your eye you will see his chest rise. Remove your mouth and turn your head away, and the chest will fall (casualty breathing out).
9. Repeat this procedure rapidly three times, to saturate the casualty's blood with oxygen, then continue the procedure regularly at the rate of about twelve times a minute. To pace yourself, here is a useful gimmick. In your mind keep repeating the following jingle at a lively rate:
   Turn head, breathe in, turn back,
   breathe out: I have got the knack.

10. If the chest fails to rise, make sure the head is titled well back and the air passage are clear, and start again.

You can continue to give the kiss of life until the causality breathes unaided. If you have been unable to summon help to send for an ambulance earlier, you can now arrange yourself for an ambulance to get the casualty to hospital.

For children and infants, use the same routine, but remember the following points:

1. Your mouth may be placed over both mouth and nose of the child.
2. Breathe out more gently into the child.

Artificial Respiration

In certain conditions the kiss of life cannot be administered, foı example, when the face is damaged to the jaw bone broken, or if the casualty has swallowed a poison which has burned the lips and mouth. The casualty must then be given artificial respiration.

1. Send for an ambulance, using any helper for the purpose.
2. Place the casualty face downwards with the arms bent so that the casualty's head rests on his hands, with the head turned to one side.
3. Kneel on one knee at the casualty's head with the foot of your opposite leg placed near the casualty's elbow.
4. Place your hands on casualty's back just below the shoulder blades or wing bones.
5. Now rock forward with your arms held straight at the elbows until your arms are vertical (upright), at the same time pressing down to compress the chest.
6. At the end of the compression allow your hands to slide sideways and outwards on to casualty's elbows.
7. Then rock backwards, lifting casualty's elbows until some resistance is felt at casualty's shoulders.
8. This movement of compression and expansion should last for two-and-a-half seconds and be repeated every five second, or twelve time a minute, until casualty starts breathing. To pace yourself, use this slightly different jingle:
   Press down, slide out, pull back
   I think I have got the knack.

For children and infants use the same routine, but using finger-tips on the shoulder blades instead of flat hands. If there was no helper to send for an ambulance earlier, you can now arrange yourself for an ambulance to get the casualty to hospital.

Acute Asthma

Asthma is the medical word for a wheezy chest. It is caused by a number of conditions of which the more common are:

1. Infection of the respiratory tract, i.e., bronchitis.
2. Allergy to pollen, dust, moulds, fur and other airborne particles.
3. Anxiety and worry.
4. Heart disease.
5. Any combination of 1 to 4.

Treatment

1. In the acute attack, allow the casualty to sit up or be propped up with pillows and cushions, in a good clean atmosphere.
2. Talk to him quietly and gently to relax him
3. Allow casualty to use inhaler if he has one, according to the dose prescribed.
4. Send for a doctor as soon as possible.
5. Do not raise dust by cleaning the room in readiness for the doctor. Do not allow flowers in the room.
6. If oxygen is available, and only if you know how to administer it, give oxygen for periods of five minutes at a time, until the doctor orders otherwise.

Heart Massage (Cardiac Compression)

Life is maintained by the continuing working of the heart and circulation of the blood. If the heart stops, then the body will die; if the blood circulation fails, then the life of the casualty is in danger. You must therefore be able to recognize when the heart has stopped and to do this you must see blue colour of the face, lips, lobes of ears, fingers and toes. The pupils of the eyes (black part) are widely dilated (enlarged). No pulsation visible in the neck or in the front of the chest. By placing your head over the front of the side of the chest you will normally be able to hear the heart beat. When the heart has stopped, you are unable to hear the heart beat.

There should be a pulse in the neck. No pulse can be felt when the heart has stopped. Sometimes the heart beat can be felt through the chest wall (left front). When the heart has stopped the heart beat cannot be felt. If therefore in unconscious casualties you see blueness and dilated pupils, feel no pulsation in the neck or chest, and hear no heart beat in the chest, you must accept that the heart has stopped and you must start immediate heart massage.

It only takes few seconds to examine a person to find whether the heart has stopped, so you are not wasting time in carrying out this routine before starting heart massage, more especially because heart massage must never be carried out on anyone whose heart has not in fact stopped.

Treatment

1. The casualty must be lying on the ground or a hard surface.
2. Turn the casualty on to his back. As if looking up to the sky.
3. Kneel at one side of the chest (the most convenient side, giving you the most room to move about).
4. Find the lower half of the breastbone (the bone to which the ribs are joined in the front of the chest).
5. Place the heel of the right hand on the lower half of the breastbone.
6. Place the left hand on top of the right.
7. With your arms straight push vertically down on the lower half of the breastbone for about 4 cm (1.5 inches) in the adult.
8. Repeat the pressure between 60–70 times a minute for adult. For children the rate is 80–90 per minute and you push chest down about 2.5 cm (1"). For infants the rate is 90–100 per minute and you push the chest down about 1.5 cm (0.5"). The rhythm of the pressure down should be as regular and even as possible. If your treatment is being given correctly you will quickly see an improvement in the colour of the casualty, i.e., the blueness will disappear and the pupils will return to normal size. You will also start to see the pulsations in the neck again. You will be able to hear the heart beat again in the chest.

If you happen to be alone with a casualty when his heart and breathing stops, you are still able to carry out heart massage. If you are fortunate enough to have a companion with you, first call an ambulance and then one of you can carry out the kiss of life and the other, the heart massage.

If the kiss of life and heart massage is really working because you and your companion have been carrying out the instructions correctly, a response in the casualty usually occurs within a few minutes of starting the operation, but this does not always follow. It may be necessary to continue the procedure for quite a long time before the casualty responds or the doctor arrives. Once the heart starts to beat again on its own, call an ambulance. You must remain with the casualty until you are able to hand him over to an ambulance attendant or doctor—in case the heart stops again and you have to start the whole process once more.

Bleeding

When there is a foreign body in the wound

This may be, for instance, a piece of glass, wood or metal.

1. Apply pressure with your finger or thumbs along the edge of the wound, leaving the foreign body in its place inside the wound. Do not remove the foreign body.
2. Apply dressings along the edge of the wound and hold them in place with a tight bandage, still leaving the foreign body in place.
3. If the wound is in an arm or leg and the bleeding profuse, lay the casualty down and raise the arm or leg above the level of the heart.
4. Arrange for an ambulance, or take casualty to hospital by car.

Bleeding nose

This is a common occurrence in the younger age groups, usually due to a small blood vessel breaking and bleeding, just inside on or other nostril. Nose bleeding is usually brought about by bangs on the nose, rubbing it excessively or through picking. It does not normally bleed for very long if the following treatment is carried out:

Treatment

1. Sit the casualty down.
2. Tilt the head slightly forward.
3. Allow the blood to drip from the nose into a bowl or basin.
4. Pinch the soft part of the nose.
5. Tell the casualty to avoid swallowing blood.

6. Bleeding usually stops within a few minutes. Casualty should rest after treatment for at least one hour. In repeated nose bleeds of this nature, the casualty should seek the advise of his doctor.

Nose bleeding in older age groups is often due to a raised blood pressure, and is frequently considered a safety valve in such cases.

Treatment

Carry out the same procedure as for younger age groups, but if bleeding does not stop in a matter of minutes and continues at a steady drip, the advice of a doctor should be sought at once. Do not plug the nose.

Coughing blood in quantity from the lungs

Coughing blood in quantity (i.e., a small cupful or more) is not a common occurrence but when it does occur it is very frightening for both the patient and relatives. It is usually the result of diseases of the lungs, such as a lung cancer or severe tuberculosis, or some form of perforating injury to the lungs.

Treatment

1. Lay the casualty down with the head and shoulders slightly raised and inclined towards the injured side.
2. Do not give any food or liquid by mouth.
3. If bleeding from the lungs is caused by a wound to the chest, then a firm padded dressing covered with a piece of polythene must be applied over the wound and secured as firmly as possible, to prevent air being sucked into the wound and so into the chest cavity, thereby causing other possible complications.
4. Send for your doctor immediately or arrange for an ambulance to take the causality to hospital.

Vomiting blood from the stomach

This is usually due to a stomach ulcer that has been bleeding. When the stomach has been filled with blood, it suddenly contracts and the casualty vomits up all the blood and this may amount to as much as a litre or more.

Treatment

1. Lay the casualty down with the feet and legs raised higher than the body.

2. Keep the casualty at a reasonable temperature. Do not overheat by applying too many blankets or hot water bottles, keep the casualty just warm, and do not let him shiver with cold.
3. Do not give any food or liquid by mouth.
4. The mouth may be washed out with water, but none must be swallowed.
5. Send immediately for a doctor, or arrange for an ambulance to take the casualty to hospital.
6. If the casualty becomes unconscious, he must immediately be turned on his side in the recovery position, but still keeping the feet and legs raised.

Unconsciousness

The loss of consciousness is always a serious sign. Unconsciousness is described as the state in which the human being will not respond in anyway to shaking, shouting or pinching. If a person who appears unconscious recovers and 'comes to' quickly when shaken, spoken to sharply, or pinched and instantly knows where he is and who he is then that person was asleep and not unconscious.

In casualties who are only just unconscious, the eyes may be moving about and when a bright light is shone into them the pupils contract. In people who are deeply unconscious, however, the eyes may be fixed as if looking straight ahead with the pupils dilated (bigger than normal); the pupils will not contract when a light is shone into them. In these conditions with the pupils dilated and the eyes fixed is one position, it usually means that the casualty is near to death. When you find a person apparently unconscious, apply the shake, shout and pinch routine. If there is no response, he is unconscious.

Causes of Unconsciousness

There is an opportunity, while waiting for the doctor or ambulance to arrive, to try and discover the cause of unconsciousness. The common causes of unconsciousness are: fainting, head injury, stroke, epilepsy—major fits of convulsions, minor fits, heart attacks, diabetes, drugs, drink, severe bleeding, acute and severe allergy, electric shock, drowning, gas poisoning.

Treatment

1. Place the casualty in the recovery position in the following manner: turn him into his back.
2. Tuck his left arm under the left buttock.
3. Place the right arm above the head.
4. Pull the body over on top of the left side.
5. Bend the right leg up to the bent position.
6. Bend the right arm into the bent position.
7. Clear away anything loose from the mouth and throat, including dentures, thus producing a clear airway so that casualty may breathe easily.
8. Ease the left arm out behind the body.
9. Now lift the head upwards and backwards to ensure that the airway is clear.

This is the left side recovery position but it may be more convenient to turn the casualty into the right-side recovery position, in which case carry out the above routine substituting right for left and vice versa.

In case where it is impossible to turn the casualty into the recovery position owing to the presence of other injuries, or his being rapped, then the maintenance of a clear airway is carried out by placing two fingers behind the angle of the jaw on both sides and pushing the jaw forward towards the nose. This will force the tongue forward and away from the back of the throat, so clearing the airway. If this simple procedure should fail to clear the airway, then open the mouth, clear any debris from it and then hold the tongue between the folds of a handkerchief and pull it forwards. The airway should then be clear.

It is important to remember that the airway must be kept clear in one of these ways until it is automatically kept clear by placing the causality in the recovery position or until a doctor or other trained person has passed a special type of breathing tube. The untrained person attempting to pass a tube ma do more harm than good to the casualty.

Do not give any food or liquid by mouth, as this will make the casualty choke and block the airway so that he cannot breathe. Send for a doctor or call for an ambulance to take the casualty to hospital. Whilst awaiting the arrival of the doctor or ambulance you must not only maintain the clear airway, but treat other injuries the casualty may have sustained.

If the casualty appears dead, i.e., if the breathing and heart appear to have just stopped, then the kiss of life and heart massage must be started immediately. A doctor or ambulance must also be summoned as soon as possible.

If the casualty is stiff from having died some time previously then leave the casualty in the position in which you find him and call a doctor and, where appropriate, the police.

The Common Faint

This occurs often in children and less frequently in adults, when they stand in one position for a long time, especially if they are not well or during very hot weather, or when they have had no food or liquids for several hours. When a person is going to faint be goes quite pale or white, with beads of perspiration on the forehead. The skin becomes cold and clammy, and he may feel he is going to be sock. Then he gently falls to the ground in a heap. If the pulse is taken at the wrist, it is usually very fast and quite weak to feel.

Provided the causality is in no further danger, as from fire or traffic, turn him into the recovery position when you will find that he will rapidly recover, in a matter of five to ten minutes. After a further short period of three to five minutes it is safe to allow him to sit up and take a glass of cold water, and then a little later on, a cup of sweet tea. If he is feeling quite normal after a rest of fifteen minutes, he may return to whatever he was originally doing. In cases of lack of food and liquids, a strong cup of sweet tea with milk and a biscuit will be helpful. This, together with a period of rest, should produce a full and normal recovery.

Head Injury

In such cases, it should be obvious that the casualty has received a blow to the skull, as for example, a car driver hitting the windscreen, a motor cyclist thrown off his motor cycle, a rider falling off his horse, a housewife falling of a ladder or downstairs. The clues are:

1. A wound is usually seen on the skull, with bleeding occurring—often quite profuse. The casualty will look pale and shocked. Pulse rate will be 90 or more in the adult.
2. The casualty will have fallen into an odd position, the airway will be restricted and therefore the breathing will be noisy.

3. Occasionally there is slight bleeding or fluid leaking from the ear or nose.
4. One pupil may be bigger than the other, with neither contracting when a light is shone into the eyes.
5. There may be bloodstained froth at the mouth.
6. The casualty may go into a conclusion (a fit) while still unconscious.

Treatment

1. Carefully supporting the head turn the casualty into the recovery position.
2. Place a loose dressing or handkerchief under the ear (untouched) so that a doctor may assess the nature of the fluid loss.
3. Control bleeding from any wound that can be seen by direct pressure and by the use of appropriate dressing and bandages. It does not apply to leakage from the ear.
4. Keep casualty in the recovery position and keep the airway clear.
5. Do not leave the casualty while he is unconscious.
6. Send for a doctor or call for an ambulance.

Stroke

This usually occurs in the middle aged to elderly, but can in rare cases occur in the young. It is due to bleeding from a burst blood vessel inside or on the surface of the brain. It is of sudden onset and usually without any warning to patient. If there is warning the casualty complains of a severe headache, gradually getting worse, followed by sudden collapse. The symptoms are:

1. Casualty often looks pale and shocked, but sometimes the face can be flushed with a purple colour.
2. The lips may be blue.
3. One side of the face may blow out with each breath whilst the opposite side will be tense and breathing will be noisy.
4. Frothing at the nose and mouth from saliva.
5. The casualty will be lip down one side of the body whilst the opposite side will be tense.
6. The pupils may be of different sizes and will not react to light; alternatively they may be equal in size and dilated.
7. The casualty may well pass urine or even have his bowels open.
8. The casualty may have a convulsion.

9. There may be aching of the muscles of the face and limbs.
10. The pulse at the wrist may be rapid and very forceful. It is easily felt.

Treatment

1. Immediately turn the casualty into the recovery position.
2. Make quite sure that airway is clear.
3. Loosen tight clothing.
4. Send for a doctor or call for an ambulance.
5. Clean up casualty after urination or bowed action.

Heart Attack

The commonest sudden heart attack is due to an obstruction of one of the coronary arteries that supply the heart muscle with blood and thus with oxygen and food substances. When a coronary artery blocks off, the muscle beyond the blockage does not receive a blood supply containing oxygen and food. The muscle therefore fails and in consequence the heart as a whole may fail and possibly stop altogether.

The casualty suffering a coronary thrombosis usually complains of a severe tight pain across the upper chest, like a tight band round the chest continually being tightened. The pain often spreads up the front of the neck, and down the inside of the left arm; occasionally it may spread down the inside of the right arm.

If the pain gets too great the heart fails to survive, the blood supply to the brain begins to fail and the casualty then becomes unconscious. The pulse is usually rapid and tends to be feeble and as the attack progresses the fingers may become blue, and finally the pupils of the eye dilate. The position in which the casualty falls will decide whether the airway will block or not. Vomiting often occurs, and this also tends to block the airway.

Treatment

1. If the casualty is sitting comfortably and is conscious then leave him sitting still and send for a doctor.
2. If the casualty collapses to the floor and becomes unconscious, turn him into the recovery position.
3. Clear the airway.
4. Constantly check that the heart is beating.

5. If the heart stops, start massage.
6. Send for a doctor or call for an ambulance.

Diabetes

Diabetes is medical condition in which the quantity of sugar in the blood rises above a certain level. In this condition a person can become unconscious, and this applies also if the quantity of sugar in the blood falls below a certain level.

In all humans the state of consciousness depends on the blood containing the correct quantity of sugar. In the untreated diabetes, if the quantity of sugar in the blood rises over a period of time (days or weeks) and when it reaches too high a level, the person becomes unconscious.

In the treated diabetic patient, taking injections of insulin, another type of unconsciousness or coma can occur. Insulin works in the body by reducing the amount of sugar circulating in the blood. If it reduces the sugar quantity too quickly or by too much, the casualty quite suddenly becomes unconscious, usually with only a short warning of a few minutes or even seconds. During this period, the casualty may have slurred speech, be irritable and obstructive. A careful search of the casualty may reveal a card or medic alert bracelet, confirming your diagnosis of diabetes. Once unconscious, he goes deeper into coma until appropriate treatment is given by a doctor.

Treatment

1. During the period of slurred speech or irritability, sugar may be given by mouth, but once the casualty becomes unconscious nothing should be given by mouth, and a doctor should be called, or the casualty sent to hospital.
2. Once the casualty has becomes unconscious he must be turned into the recovery position and the airway cleared of any obstruction.
3. Do not leave the casualty alone while he is unconscious.

Drug

A large proportion of drugs and medicines when taken in too large quantity at one time will produce a state of unconsciousness. This applies equally to drugs prescribed by doctor or obtained through a drug pusher.

Treatment (unconscious)

1. Turn casualty into the recovery position.
2. Clear his airway.
3. Call for a doctor and ambulance.
4. A close watch must be kept on breathing and heartbeat. If either or both fail, the kiss of life and/or heart massage must be started immediately.
5. Do not remove or destroy the empty bottles in which the tablets or medicine were contained, and do not remove any vomit from around the casualty. The bottles and specimens of vomit should be sent to the hospital for testing in the laboratory.
6. If the person is obviously dead, then you must also send for the police and do not touch anything in the room where the person is lying.

Treatment (conscious)

1. If the casualty has taken drugs and is still conscious, then you must endeavour to keep him conscious by talking to him.
2. Arrange for urgent admission to hospital.
3. Again the empty bottles of any vomit must be kept for analysis.
4. Do not give large quantities of fluid such as water or an emetic; and do not make the casualty vomit to get rid of the drug. It is better to get a doctor or get the casualty to hospital in as short a time as possible.

Electric Shock

This is usually easy to identify, as the casualty will be lying unconscious near an electrical appliance or cable.

Treatment

1. Before touching the casualty remember to switch off the electric supply.
2. If the casualty is breathing, turn him into the recovery position.
3. If the casualty has stopped breathing, you must start the kiss of life and heart massage immediately.
4. Send for a doctor or ambulance.

Drowning: Treatment

1. Clear the airway and determine whether casualty is breathing and the heart pumping.
2. If the heart and breathing have stopped, then you must immediately start the Kiss of Life and heart massage.
3. If the casualty is just unconscious, then once removed from the water, he should be placed in the recovery position.
4. A doctor or an ambulance should be sent for immediately.

Burns and Scalds

Burns and scalds can have distressing effects, such as scarring, deformity and mental trauma; these effects can all be long-lasting, and sometimes even permanent. Correct, careful and prompt treatment of deep burns is therefore essential.

Burns occur when the body is in contact with, or too close to, dry heat and strong chemicals and among the many frequent causes are:

1. Kitchen utensils such as baking tins, oven shelves and pan handles.
2. Modern electrical equipment, including kettles, hotplates and irons.
3. Accidental fires from open grates, gas and electric fires.
4. Clothing and other articles accidentally set alight.
5. Excessive sun and wind.
6. Accidents wit.h ropes.

Because of their character, burns are most often sustained by the exposed parts of the body, particularly the hands, wrists and head. Scalds, on the other hand, occur when the body is in contact with moist heat, such as steam or hot water, fats or oils, and other hot liquids. But there the differences end for our purposes, because the resulting effect on the skin is much the same. A 'burn' means a burn or a scald. The damage from burns can range from a mere reddening of the affected skin to blister formation and, in more serious cases, to actual destruction of the tissues. In hospital language, burns are described as being superficial of deep, depending on the depth of the damage. Superficial burns are in fact more painful. But in first aid it is not the depth, but the surface area of the burn, by which its seriousness is measured.

Most burns happen in the home, so that is where they have to be treated; and as most home accidents take place in the kitchen, the kitchen is probably the best room in which to treat casualties. The groups at the greatest risk are the elderly, the physically handicapped, and children—especially toddlers. All burns to children and the elderly must be taken seriously.

Treatment

1. Immerse the injured part in cold water. This may be done using a bucket or washing up bowl, the kitchen sink, or simply holding the burn under a gently running cold tap. The burn should be immersed in cold water for about fifteen minutes or until the pain has stopped. If it is difficult to immerse the injury (on the face, for instance), soak a clean tea cloth or any other clean soft material in cold water and apply it to the injury as a compress. Do not rub the surface of the burn. This treatment will take some of the heat out of the tissues and prevent further damage, reddening, blistering and pain.
2. Remove rings, bracelets, shoes and tight fitting articles as soon as possible after injury, as swelling may develop making it difficult to remove them later.
3. Small superficial burns should be carefully patted dry once pain has stopped, and then covered with a dressing. Larger areas or deep burns when removed from the water should be covered lightly with clean, recently laundered, non fluffy material.
4. Send for a doctor or call for am ambulance.
5. Any burn larger than a postage stamp (2 × 2½ cm) must be seen by a doctor, who should be summoned after you have applied cooling treatment.
6. When a large area is damaged, requiring hospital care, ice may be packed in a towel and applied to the injury during the journey.
7. It is essential to cover up burnt tissue to prevent infection, which thrives on burn skin. This also reduces the anxiety of the casualty, who can no longer see the burn. Table clothes or sheets (not nylon) are excellent for covering the body. The covering should be held in place lightly.
8. While waiting for doctor or ambulance, reassure and comfort casualty. Pick up a child and cuddle.

References

Andrews, S. (2007) *Hotel Housekeeping Training Manual*. Tata McGraw Hill Publishing Co. Ltd., New Delhi.

Branson, J. and M. Lennox. (1988) *Hotel, Hostel and Hospital Housekeeping*. 5th Edition, McGraw Hill, New York.

Branson, J. and M. Lennox. (1998) *Incorporating the Second Edition of Hotel Housekeeping*. Arnold Heinemann, New Delhi.

David, J. (2005) *Textbook of Hotel Management*. Anmol Publications Pvt. Ltd., New Delhi.

Isaac Mary (1976) *Towards Better Homes*. Allahabad Saint Paul Society, Allahabad.

Kamra, Krishna, Robert Mill and S. Kaushil. (2000) *Hospitality: Operations and Management*. Wheeler Publishing, Allahabad.

5

Changes in Clothing Interest of Women during Old Age

A Study

SHIVANI VERMA AND VANDANA R. CHAUHAN

Clothes not only serve a utilitarian purpose of covering the body, but are also used with special effect to enhance the beauty and elegance of an individual.

Ever since primitive people began to adorn their naked bodies with coloured clays, men and women have been occupying themselves more or less with attaining, enhancing and preserving of external beauty in themselves.

We are all aware of the increasing importance of clothes in our day-to-day life. As rightly said by Marilyn. J. Horn throughout recorded history, clothing along with food and shelter has been one of the primary needs of mankind. The ways in which individuals and families have fulfilled this need over the years provide ample evidence that the pattern of production, distribution, and consumption of clothing, figure largely in the economic development of a country. Moreover, clothing is not only of intimate concern to the individual in terms of one's physical and psychological well-being, but it reflects the values, the conditions, and the developments of society as a whole.

Since ages women have been known to be interested in clothing. Interest in clothes varies from person to person and within the same person. It can be different during different stages in the life span.

Every stage in one's life cycle brings new sets of values, attitudes and interests. One has to also adjust to the changes in the attitudes of others towards him/her.

Old age is the last stage in the life span. It begins from 60 years.

Certain changes are natural accompaniment of what is commonly known as "ageing". They affect the physical as well as the mental structure and functioning of an individual.

The development tasks of old age include:

- Adjusting to decreasing physical strength and health.
- Adjusting to retirement and reduced income.
- Adjusting to death of spouse.
- Establishing an explicit affiliation with members of one's age group.
- Establishing satisfactory physical living arrangements.
- Adapting to social roles in a flexible way.

Old age is a time of life beset by particular and acute problems which may also stem from role expectations.

Interest in clothes to some extent depends how socially active the elderly are, partly on the economic status, and partly how willing they are to accept the fact that they are growing old and must adjust to it. Some elderly people continue to wear styles they wore earlier and refuse to dress according to current fashion, even when it means that they must have their garments made to order.

Other older people by contrast are very fashion conscious and may choose clothes that are designed for those young enough to be their children or even their grandchildren. They are rebelling against old age and are trying to convince themselves and others that they are younger than they really are.

Limited incomes prevent many elderly people from having as great as interest in their clothes and appearance as they might otherwise have.

Older people's interest in clothing is also affected by the difficulty they have in finding ready-made clothes that are stylish and yet fit their ageing figures.

The older individual is still interested in clothing and is motivated to look attractive to others. The need to make new friends may be even greater than in earlier years because of the loss of old friends; thus the older person wishes to have stylish clothes and not to be set apart in a separate group by different clothing.

The problem in dressing attractively are greater than they are for young persons. In the first place, the older individuals are often retired and thus are living on a reduced income. This is partially revealed by the fact that older women tends to be less active socially and so has less need for clothes.

There are physical changes in the body with advancing age which have implications on clothing.

Thus clothes have been the fascination to enhance a person's appearance as well as to boost morale, regardless of age. It satisfies functional, social and aesthetic need of people of all ages. It has a social and psychological impact.

Objectives of the Study

The study was conducted in April 1997 on "The Changes in Clothing Interest During Different Stages in Women's Life". The focus, here, in this article in on clothing interest of women during old age.

The objectives of the study were:

1. To study the physiological, psychological and sociological characteristics pertaining to old age.
2. To study and compare the interest in clothing during different stages of women's life.
3. To study the relationship of clothing interest to qualification, income level, marital status and family type, i.e., joint or nuclear.
4. To study the effect of clothing interest on old women's self-esteem/self-concept, if any.

Thus the investigators felt that this study would further enhance the growing knowledge in the field of clothing behaviour in relation to the older women.

Hypotheses

1. With the increase in age, clothing interest decreases.
2. There is no correlation between the variables clothing interest and qualification, clothing interest and marital status, clothing interest and monthly income, clothing interest and family type, for old age.
3. There is no correlation between the variables clothing interest and self-esteem/self-concept, for old age.

Limitations

1. The study was limited to women in their adolescence, early adulthood, middle years and old age. In this article, only old age has been considered.
2. The study was limited to 200 respondents (50 in each category) comprising of the staff, students and their family members of the Faculty of Home Science, M.S. University of Baroda, Vadodara. In this article, only old age has been considered.

Methodology

Total sample size was 50 respondents, who were old. Quota sampling procedure, followed by selection of the samples randomly was followed.

A questionnaire was formulated. Content validity was done. Suggested alterations were made as per the suggestions given by a panel of judges, comprising of psychologists and home scientists. A pilot study was first conducted. Then the questionnaire was actually executed on the old women. The data was coded and then presented and statistically analysed.

Results

The demographic variables of older women have been presented in Table 1.

Graph 1 *Represents the frequency distribution of the income level of old age women showing the monthly income of the family, amounts per month spent on family clothing and amount per month spent on one's own clothing, i.e., old age women*

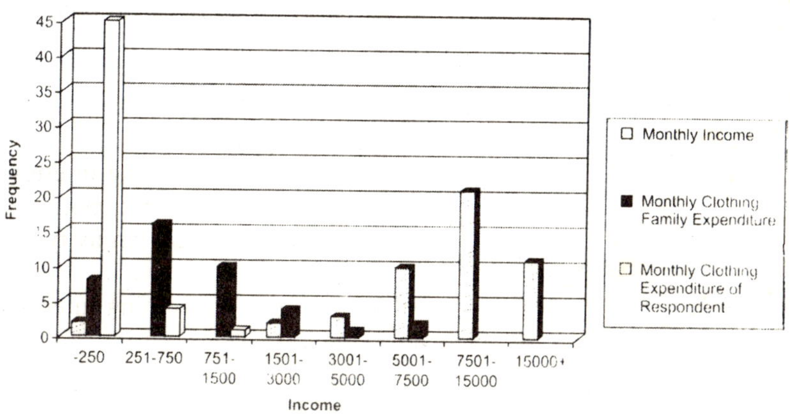

Table 1 *Frequency Distribution of Demographic Variables of Old Age Women*

Frequency	Qualificational Level			Occupational Status		Marital Status				Type of Family		
	Up to SSC	Above SSC and under-graduate	Graduate and post-graduate	Working	House Wife	Single	Married	Widow	Divorced	Nuclear	Joint	Single
0	–	–	–	2	–	1	–	–	–	–	–	1
5	–	–		–	–	–	–	–	–	–	–	–
10	–	–	7	–	–	–	–	–	–	9	–	–
15	–	–	–	–	–	–	–	–	–	–	–	–
20	–	–	–	–	–	–	–	–	–	–	–	–
25	–	–	–	–	–	–	24	25	–	–	–	–
30	–	–	–	–	–	–	–	–	–	–	–	–
35	–	–	–	–	–	–	–	–	–	–	–	–
40	–	–	–	–	–	–	–	–	–	–	40	–
45	43	–	–	–	–	–	–	–	–	–	–	–
50	–	–	–	–	48	–	–	–	–	–	–	–

Pie Diagram 1

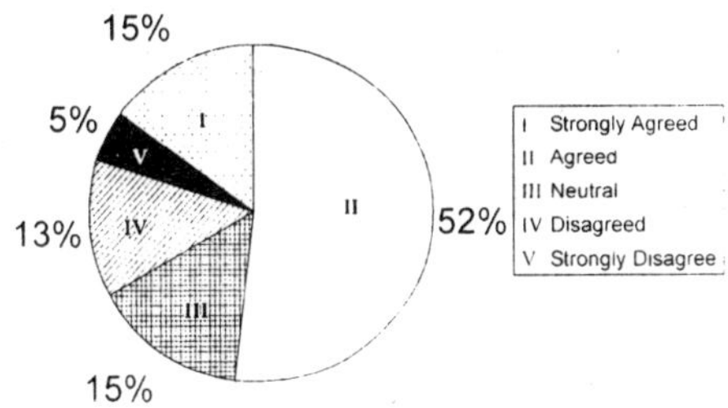

The responses to the positive statements pertaining to old age have been presented in Pie Diagram 1.

It indicates that 15 per cent of the respondents strongly agreed to them, 52 per cent agreed, 15 per cent were neutral, 13 per cent disagreed and 5 per cent strongly disagreed. Thus from the above responses, certain characteristics of old age to which majority agreed to were:

- Many old women show little interest in how they look.
- As grown up children become increasingly involved in their own affairs, the elderly can count less and less on their companionship.
- Inclination towards religion is maximum during old age.
- Meeting social and civic obligations is difficult for many old ladies as their health fails and as their income is reduced by retirement.
- It is expected that an old lady will play a decreasingly less active role in social affairs.
- Old age is a period when people "move away" from previous more desirable periods or times of "usefulness".
- Old age is an age of illness, loneliness and loss of strength.
- Feeling unwanted and useless, an elderly lady develops feelings of inferiority and resentment.
- Mental decline is maximum in old age.
- The elderly or aged people have minority group status.
- Poor adjustment is characteristic of old age.
- Because of unfavourable social attitudes towards the elderly that are reflected in the way the social group treats them, it is not surprising that many elderly people develop unfavourable self-concepts.

The responses to the negative statements pertaining to old age women have been presented in Pie Diagram 2.

Pie Diagram 2

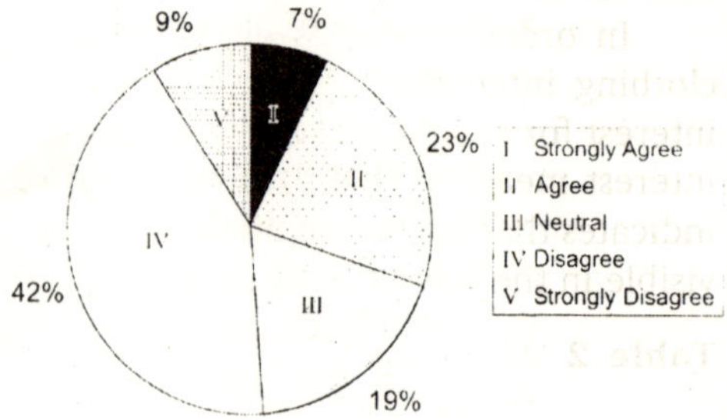

It indicates that 7 per cent of the respondents strongly agreed to them, 23 per cent agreed, 19 per cent were neutral, 42 per cent disagreed and 9 per cent strongly disagreed. Thus, from the above responses, it was seen that certain characteristics of old age to which majority disagreed were:

- There is no social disengagement during old age.
- Even though an elderly women's interest in self increases and she remain preoccupied with herself, she never becomes ego-centric and self-centred.
- Because an elderly cannot compete with young people in areas where highly valued traits are needed, the social attitude towards them are unfavourable.
- Older women, who spend their younger years mainly in home, are never careful of their appearance in old age just as they were when young.
- During old age, there are least physical, psychological and lifestyle changes and also least changes in interest.
- There are minimum physical, psychological, personal and social hazards in old age.

Statistical Analysis of Clothing Interests

Responses to all the positive statements were put on a scale from 5 to 1 and all the negative on 1 to 5.

For each of the age group, mean clothing interest measure of the respondents was calculated by first of all adding up the scores for both the positive and the negative statements and then dividing by the number of the statements and the number of the respondents in each group (i.e., 50).

This study was carried out to study the changes in clothing interest during different stages of women's life. The focus here in this research article is on old age. The measure of clothing interest of the respondents belonging to different age groups have been mentioned here for comparison.

In order to test the hypothesis that with the increase in age, clothing interest decreases, a mean measure, or score of clothing interest for each of the age groups were taken. The average clothing interest measure or scores has been represented in Table 2, which indicates that as the age increases, clothing interest decreases. This is visible in the score for old age, i.e., 2.92.

Table 2 *Measure of Clothing Interest of the Respondents Belonging to Different Age Groups*

Age Groups	*Measure of Clothing Interest*
Adolescence	3.62
Early Adulthood	3.61
Middle Age	3.43
Old Age	2.92

Statistical analysis of the attitude statements (measure of clothing interest) with section I, i.e., demographic variables

Correlation Coefficient between the variables clothing interest and qualification, clothing interest and monthly income and clothing interest and family type, i.e., joint or nuclear was found out for old age.

It was observed that correlation coefficient between clothing interest and qualification in case of old age was 0.64.

In order to make it more interesting and meaningful, the investigator investigated the minimum correlation coefficient that would be there in the population.

Considering the hypothesis H1: Population correlation coefficient between the variables clothing interest and qualification among old age is 0.65 (say).

Since Z equals to 0.758 and M equals to 0.775 and standard deviation equals to 0.15 under the test statistic,

$U = Z–M/\sqrt{N–3} \sim N(0,1) = -0.106$

Since $|U|$ is less than 1.96 it is not significant at 5 per cent level of significance. Hence, the hypothesis H1 may be accepted. Therefore, the sample may be regarded as coming from the population with correlation coefficient as 0.60.

It was observed that the correlation coefficient between the variables clothing interest and marital status in case of old age was 0.32.

Considering the hypothesis H2: Population Correlation Coefficient between the variables clothing interest and marital status among old age women is 0.30 (say).

Since, Z equals to 0.332 and M equals to 0.301 and standard deviation equals to 0.15 under the test statistic,

$U = (Z–M)/\sqrt{N–3} \sim N(0, 1) = 0.152.$

Since |U| is less than 1.96 it is not significant at 5 per cent level of significance. Hence, the hypothesis H2 may be accepted. Therefore, the sample may be regarded as coming from the population with correlation coefficient as 0.030.

It was observed that the correlation coefficient between the variables clothing interest and monthly income of the family in case of old age was 0.68.

Considering the hypothesis H3: Population correlation coefficient between the variables clothing interest and monthly income of the family among old age respondents is 0.70 (say).

Since, Z equals to 0.829 and M equals to 0.867 and standard deviation equals to 0.15 under the test statistic,

$U = (Z–M)/\sqrt{N–3} \sim N(0, 1) = –0.262.$

Since |U| is less than 1.96 it is not significant at 5 per cent level of significance. Hence, the hypothesis H3 may be accepted. Therefore, the sample may be regarded as coming from the population with correlation coefficient as 0.70.

It was observed that the correlation coefficient between the variables clothing interest and the type of family in case of old age was 0.39.

Considering the hypothesis H4: Population correlation coefficient between the variables clothing interest and family type among old age is 0.40 (say).

Since, Z equals to 0.412 and M equals to 0.424 and standard deviation equals to 0.15 under the test statistic,

$U = (Z–M)/\sqrt{N–3} \sim N(0, 1) = –0.081.$

Since |U| is less than 1.96 it is not significant at 5 per cent level of significance. Hence the hypothesis H4 may be accepted. Therefore, the sample may be regarded as coming from the population with correlation coefficient as 0.40.

Thus, it has been accepted that the variables, namely, clothing interest and qualification, clothing interest and marital status, clothing interest and monthly income of the family and clothing interest and type of family were correlated. However, it was observed that no variable independent of the others acted upon clothing interest. A interest one has in clothing depends on a complex mix of several variable acting upon it.

Statistical analysis of the attitude statements, for the measure of clothing interest in section III of the questionnaire with measure of self-esteem/self-concept in section IV of the questionnaire

The attitude statements of section III comprised of a measure of clothing interest. Section IV comprised of statements to measure an individual's self-esteem/self-concept.

To calculate the mean measure of clothing interest and self-esteem/self-concept, responses to all the positive and negative statements were scored by the investigator. All the positive statements were put on a scale from 5 to 1 and all the negative statements on a scale from 1 to 5. Scores of the positive statements were added up and then divided by the number of respondents (i.e., 50).

Table 3 represents the mean scores of self-esteem/self-concept for each of the four age groups.

Table 3 *Measure of Self-esteem/Self-concept of the Respondents Belonging to Different Age Groups*

Age Groups	*Measure of Self-esteem/Self-concept*
Adolescence	2.59
Early Adulthood	2.74
Middle Age	2.81
Old Age	3.06

It is evident from Table 3, that the mean measure for self-concept was highest in old age. It indicates that as the age increases self-esteem/self-concept also increases. This is visible in the score for old age, i.e., 3.06

Hypothesis III

In order to test the hypothesis that population correlation coefficient between the variable clothing and self-esteem/self-concept is zero for old age, t-test was applied. In order to test the significance from an uncorrelated bivariate normal universe, t-test was used if 'r' is the observed correlation coefficient in a sample of 'n' pairs of observations from bivariate normal population than Fisher's test says that considering the null hypothesis H0: Population Correlation Coefficient is zero then the test statistics $t = [r/\sqrt{1 - r^2})] \times (\sqrt{n\text{-}2})$ follows.

If the values of t comes out to be non-significant H0 would be rejected at the level of significance adopted and concluded that population Correlation is not 'zero'. If t comes out to be significant then H0 may be accepted and it would be concluded that the variation may be regarded as uncorrelated to the universe.

Considering the hypothesis: Population Coefficient between the variables Clothing Interest and self-esteem/self-concept of old age is zero.

Under H, $t = [r/\sqrt{1 - r^2})] \times (\sqrt{n\text{-}2})$

$= [0.05/\sqrt{1 - 0.05^2})] \times (\sqrt{50\text{-}2})$

$= 0.35$

Since t tabulated, i.e., 1.96 was greater that t calculated at 5 per cent level of significance and 48 d.f. hypothesis was accepted and it was concluded that there was no correlation between the variables clothing interest and self-esteem/self-concept in old age respondents.

Thus, from the above hypothesis testing discussion, it was observed that in case of old age respondents and 48 clothing interest and self-esteem/self-concept showed no correlation at 5 per cent level of significance and 48 d.f.

It can be concluded from this research that the clothing interest varied during old age.

Select References

Ambron, S.A. and D. Brodzinsby. (1979) *Life Span Development*. Halt, Rinehart and Winston, United States of America, p. 339, 420, 465, 555.

Chambers, H.G. and V. Moulton. (1961) *Clothing Selection*. J.B. Lippincott and Co., Philadelphia, pp. 29–32.

Dikey, L.E. (1967) Projection of Self-Esteem, Security-Insecurity and to Selected Clothing Behaviours, Unpublished Doctoral Thesis, Pennsylvania State University, p. 1, 2, 6, 7, 11, 12, 14, 15.

Ebeling, M. and M.L. Rosencranz. (1961) "Social and Personal Aspects of Clothing for Older Women". *Journal of Home Economics*, Vol. 56, No. 6, pp. 464–465.

Grover, Rashmi. (1973) A Study of Self-Esteem, Security-Insecurity and Clothing Interest of the Students of the Faculty of Home Science, Baroda, Unpublished Master's Dissertation, Department of Clothing and Textiles, Faculty of Home Science, M S University of Baroda, p. 1, 4, 5, 7, 11.

Klasen, M.G. (1967) Self-Esteem and its Relationship to Clothing, Master's Dissertation, Michigan State University, Michigan.

Rosencranz, Mary L.L. (1949) "A Study of Women's Interest in Clothing". *Journal of Home Economics*, pp. 460–462.

Workman, J.E. and Kim K.P. Johnson. (1993) "The Effect of Three Status Characteristics on Rating of an Elderly Male and an Elderly Female: Social Variable". *Journal* of *Home Economics*, Vol. 21, No. 3, pp. 261–279.

6

Ergonomically Designed Toilet Chair

A Remedy to Avoid Accidents Among Old Age People

NIRMAL KAUR AND PROMILA SHARMA

It is well known that the world's population is ageing, with more developed regions leading the process, because of increasing survival to older ages as well as smaller numbers of births (United Nations Population Division, 1998 revision). Consequently, the support of this ever expanding elderly population has become of increasing concern. Approximately 20 per cent of people aged 70 years or older, and 50 per cent of people aged 85 and over, experienced difficulties in such basic activities of daily living as bathing, dressing and toileting. Changes in body composition are well known to occur with old age, but there is limited knowledge of the normal values rate of changes in anthropometric indices of body composition or the distribution of these changes in the elderly. The anthropometric standards derived from adult population may not be appropriate for the elderly because of body composition changes occurring during ageing. Specific anthropometric reference data for the elderly are necessary, before designing any kind of product or furniture or similar related equipment.

Nowadays the knee problem is very common among third age people who creates hindrance in using Indian toilet seat because of their problem to sit down on the feet and folding their knees. Thus, to avoid it seat height should be 20"–24" that will give better leverage in regaining a standing position and the fall and slip injuries can be checked which are associated with this knee problem as it is quoted by Heikkinen et al. (2002) that more than one-third of adults' of ages 65 years and older fall each year.

Materials and Methods

Experimental design was planned to study eight anthropometric measurements, necessary for designing of toilet chair through Computer Aided Design (CAD). The whole list of males and females of old age people of Pantnagar and Rudrapur block was made and than out of that list, 100 old age people each from both the blocks were chosen using simple random sampling without replacement, out of which 50 per cent were male and 50 per cent were female, thus altogether making total size of 200 people of third age. Different scientific instruments used for collection of experimental data were anthropometric rods, weighing balance and grip dynamometer. For designing of toilet chair 5th, 50th and 95th percentile values were calculated.

I. 5th Percentile

It is used to measure the minimum requirement with regard to height, length and width, etc.

II. 50th Percentile

It is used to measure the average requirement with regard to height, length and width, etc.

III. 95th Percentile

It is used to measure the maximum requirement with regard to height, length and width, etc.

$$Pp = 1 + \frac{PN - F}{fp} \times i$$

where,

Pp = required percentile rank

1 = Lowest value of the class interval where Pp falls

PN = Cumulative frequency in relation to the Pp point

F = Cumulative frequency below the lowest value of Pp class

fp = actual frequency of Pp class

i = class interval score

Results and Discussion

The anthropometric measurements of third age people were taken and on the bases of that the total value was calculated as shown in Table 1, for the designing of toilet chair. It was found by the correlation coefficient that there was a significant relationship among the

Table 1 *Anthropometric Measurements of Old Age People*

Sitting Measurement	*Male (cm)*					*Female (cm)*					*Total (cm)*				
	M	*SD*	*5th*	*50th*	*95th*	*M*	*SD*	*5th*	*50th*	*95th*	*M*	*SD*	*5th*	*50th*	*95th*
Sitting Height*	80	4.9	72	80.5	8.6	75.5	3.0	71	76	80	78	4.9	71	77	86
Sitting Shoulder Height*	55	3.7	51	54	61	54	3.0	50	53	59	54	3.5	50	54	61
Buttock Popliteal Length	45	3.7	40	45	53	44	3.1	39.5	44	49	44	3.4	38.5	44.5	50
Popliteal Height*	44	2.6	40	44	49	41	4.8	36	42	46	42	4.1	39	43	46
Elbow Rest Height*	21	3.5	16	21	26	20	3.5	15	20	25	20	3.5	15	21	26
Hip Breadth*	38	4.0	34	37	44	38	4.4	30	37.5	43.5	38	4.2	33	37	44
Hand Length*	17	1.3	15.5	17.5	19	17	1.2	15.5	17	19	17	1.2	16	17	19
Grip Strength	16	10.4	0	15	31	12	9.6	0	9	31	13	10.2	0	11	31

* Significant relationship.

Different Views and Parts of the Toilet Chair

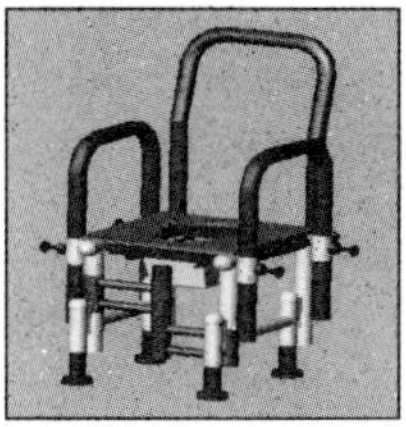
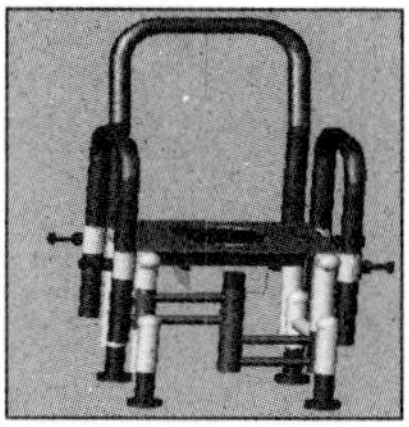

Front view of toilet chair

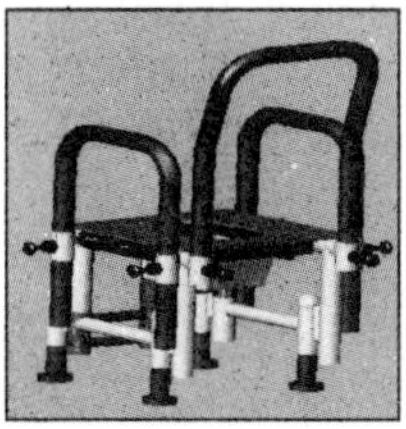

Side view of toilet chair

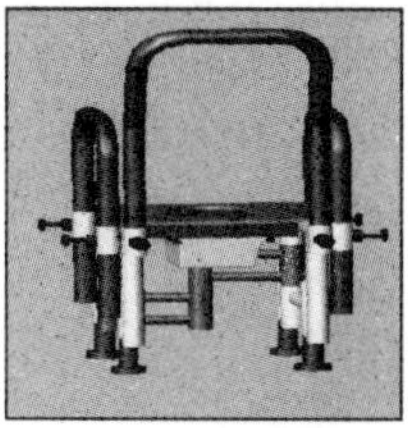

Back view of toilet chair

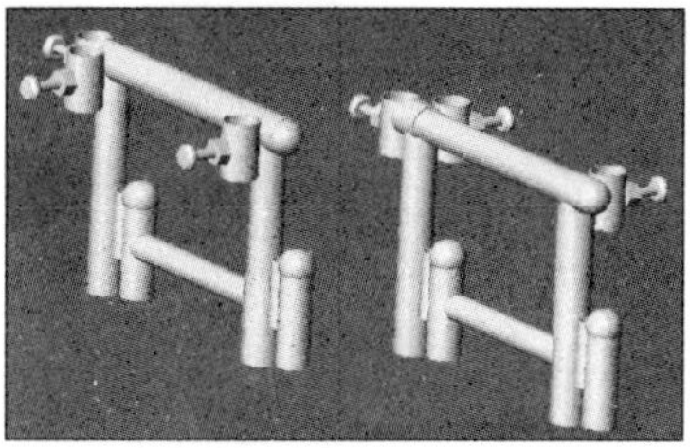

Legs of toilet chair

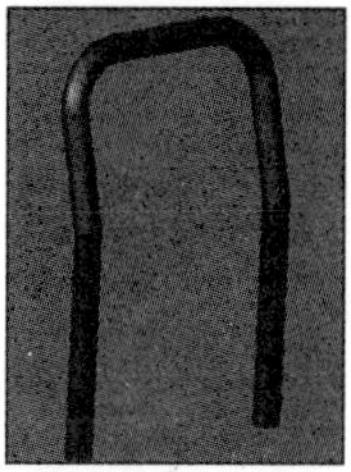

Backrest rod of toilet chair

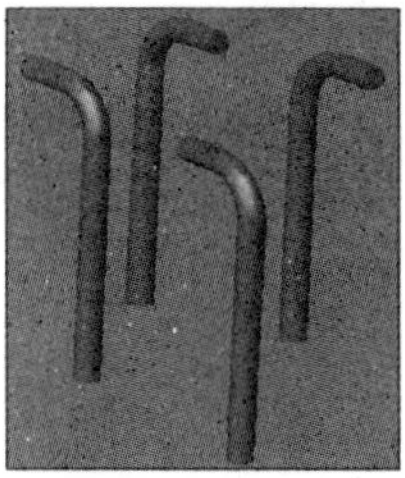

Handrest rods of toilet chair

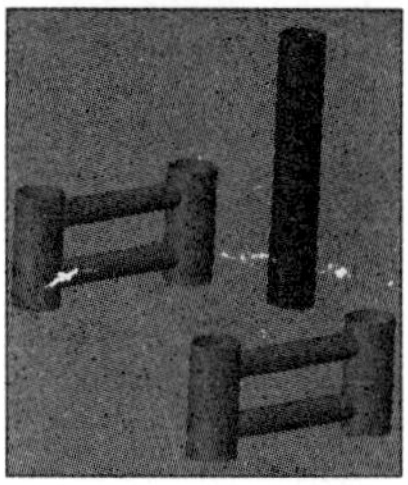

Assembled parts of toilet chair

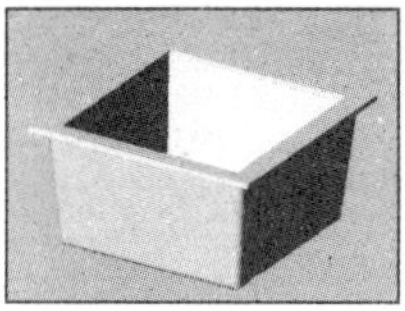

Pan of toilet chair

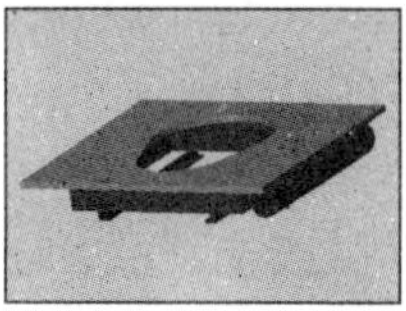

Seat plate of toilet chair

dimensions of males and females of third age. It can be seen from Table 2 that for seat height all the three values of 5th percentile, 50th percentile and 95th percentile was taken so that all kinds of people, i.e., shortest, average and tallest can be easily accommodate. For seat width 95th percentile and for seat depth 5th percentile value was taken. In handrest and backrest 95th percentile was taken as well as the provision of adjustment was given. As the old age people were having the problem of support, in the front, support handle was also given in the toilet chair. The weight of the toilet chair was made as per the 50th percentile value of the grip strength of old age people.

On the basis of these data the design of toilet chair was developed through CAD.

Table 2 *Dimensions for Designing of Toilet Chair for the Old Age People*

Measurements	*5th Percentile*	*50th Percentile*	*95th Percentile*
Sitting Height (for extending backrest height)	—	—	86 cm
Sitting Shoulder Height (for backrest height)	—	—	61 cm
Buttock Popliteal Length (for seat depth)	38.5 cm	—	—
Popliteal Height (for seat height)	39 cm	43 cm	46 cm
Elbow Rest Height (for hand rest height)	15 cm	21 cm	26 cm
Hip Breadth (for seat width)	—	—	44 cm
Hand Length (for circumference)	16 cm	—	—
Grip Strength (for weight of chair)	—	10 kg	—

Table 3 *Age and Sex Wise Occurrence of Accidents*

Criteria	*60–65 Years*		*65–70 Years*		*Total*		*Chi-square Values*
	M	*F*	*M*	*F*	*M*	*F*	
Fall due to standing after sitting	15 (15)	18 (18)	26 (26)	44 (44)	41 (20.5)	62 (31)	0.6,466 NS
Fall due to no support	10 (10)	19 (19)	25 (25)	30 (30)	35 (17.5)	49 (24.5)	0.9,404 NS
Fall due to slippery ness	4 (4)	7 (7)	8 (8)	11 (11)	12 (6)	18 (9)	0.0,956 NS
Total	29	44	59	85	88	129	

Figures in parentheses represent percentage.

Home injuries occur as a result of falls, slips and most of these accidents are considered preventable. Table 3 revealed that age and sexwise distribution of total number of accidents among the people of third age. It was found that all accidents due to fall related to use of Indian toilet were more in case of females rather than males of third age, which results in injuries and it can be seen in the table that it was increasing with the increase in the age.

Table 4 *Extent of Satisfaction Derived by Third Age People from Ergonomically Designed Toilet Chair*

Description	*Highly Satis- fied = 3*	*Satis- fied = 2*	*Not Satisfied = 1*	*Total Score*	*Mean Score*
Height of chair	14 (70)	6 (30)	—	54	2.7
Weight of chair	3 (15)	12 (60)	5 (25)	38	1.9
Width of chair	15 (75)	5 (25)	—	55	2.75
Depth of chair	15 (75)	5 (25)	—	55	2.75
Height of handrest	20 (100)	—	—	60	3
Supporting handle	13 (65)	7 (35)	—	53	2.65
Operation of assembling	5 (25)	13 (65)	2 (10)	43	2.15
Removal of pan	5 (25)	12 (60)	3 (15)	42	2.1
Able to carry chair	3 (15)	9 (45)	8 (40)	35	1.75
Material of toilet chair	15 (75)	5 (25)	—	55	2.75
Material of seat plate	4 (20)	11 (55)	5 (25)	39	1.95
Material of backrest	5 (25)	15 (75)	—	45	2.25
Material of handrest	14 (70)	6 (30)	—	54	2.7
Comfortableness	14 (70)	6 (30)	—	54	2.7
Cost of chair	5 (25)	10 (50)	5 (25)	40	2.0

Figures in parentheses represent percentage.

Table 5 *Distribution of Third Age People by their Scores on Extent of Satisfaction Derived*

Score	*Range*	*Third Age People*
0–15	Low	2 (10)
15–30	Moderate	6 (30)
30–45	High	12 (60)

The satisfaction among old age people was calculated about the ergonomically designed chair. Table 5 showed that 60 per cent people of third age were found to be in high level range, while 30 per cent in moderate range of satisfaction level. There were 10 per cent people who were in the range of low level of satisfaction

Conclusion

As the design of toilet chair was made by using anthropometric data of old age people, it is expected that the problem among these group can be solved to some extent and we will be able to avoid the cases of accidents during the use of different kinds of toilets by these people.

References

Heikkinen, R.L., S. Berg, K. Avlund and T. Tormakangas. (2002) "Depressed Mood: Changes during a Five-year Follow-up in 75 year-old Men and Women in Three Nordic Localities". *Aging Clin. Exp. Res.*, 14 (Suppl. 3), pp. 16–27.

U.S. Bureau of the Census. (1996) Population Projections of the United States by Age, Sex, Race and Hispanic Origin: 1995–2050. Current Population Reports, US Government Printing Office, Washington DC, pp. 25–1130.

7

Elderly and Recreation

BABITA SHUKLA

Recreation is viewed here as any activity or pursuit which is voluntarily chosen by the participant within his leisure time, with the primary motivation of achieving personal pleasure, and with a minimum of other hoped-for goals or compulsions surrounding it. Clearly when we refer to recreation as activity carried on for its own sake, it is difficult to ignore all the varied pressures one faces in making leisure choice. One may have feeling of family responsibility in planning certain leisure activities, such as picnic or outings, and undoubtedly some who participate in physical recreation do so with a dutiful sense of 'keeping fit' in recognizing that a number of such extrinsic purposes or pressures may surround any leisure activity, it is necessary to measure the degree of challenge within the activity itself and the amount of personal enjoyment received by the participant, in order to determine whether it truly deserves the name of recreation.

A term which has frequently been associated with recreation is 'play'. This may refer to recreational pursuits in general, as in the phrase 'the world of play'. It may also be used to describe the specific act of carrying on certain recreational activities they are played.

In considering recreation, an extremely broad range of possible characteristics must be recognized:

- What one person views as recreational may not be so for another person. Indeed, an activity may be recreational for an individual at a given time and place, and not in another.

- Recreation may be the most trivial and unimportant of pursuits, or it may involve serious dedication and be on the highest level of purpose and intensity.
- Recreation may involve a single casual episode, or it may continue as a deeply satisfying activity throughout a lifetime.
- Recreation may be passive, not the physically and mentally, or may involve extremely active participation on a variety of levels.
- Recreation may be completely solitary; it may also involve small groups or large masses of people.
- Recreation may be socially constructive and serve important personal and social needs, or it may represent degrading, time-wasting, or even anti-social or criminal forms of activity.

Recognizing that one's leisure time may be spent in a variety of ways, let us examine those forms of leisure activity that are voluntarily chosen and are pleasurable therefore, viewed as recreation. These may be classified in two broad categories:

Private Recreation

This includes the kind of activity which is carried on by individuals or families, either within the home or neighbourhood, or in trips, or in other settings which require no formal sponsorship or organization.

Public Recreation

A host of somewhat more formal and structured recreational activities are sponsored by governmental agencies, or by voluntary semi-public organization. As examples, one might include the various kinds of sports or cultural activities offered by municipal recreation departments: outdoor activities and other recreational programme.

Commercial recreation

This consists of the kinds of recreational activities offered to the public at large by the mass media, television, radio, magazines, films, etc.

Importance of Recreational Activities

The source of the term 'recreation' was originally the Latin recreation, meaning to restore or refresh, extended, this means that an activity which restores one to a state of vigour and alertness from a state of weakness or exhaustion is recreational. Recreation depends for its social justification upon work. It was seen as a reward for work well done, and it intended to prepare the individual for further work.

Today, of course, as work has become less labourious and demanding, this traditional view of the function of recreation has become less widely accepted. It is no longer necessary to see it in relation to economically productive activity; it is productive and valuable in its own right.

Personal Values of Recreation

Probably the most important single reason why people take part in recreational experience is that it brings a direct measure of happiness to them. The direct outcomes of successful recreation experience for the individual may be listed under the following headings:

Social Outcomes

The social outcomes and values of recreational experience are important for those of all ages, but particularly so for young people. It is in the peer group, engaging in play activities, that children begin to develop social competence. For adolescents and adults as well, a wide variety of satisfying group contacts, in which the individual relates effectively to others, shares their concerns and needs, and is accepted by them as a human being, is essential to social growth.

Creative Outcomes

Recreation also permits the individual to be himself and to explore his own, special creative talents. This is particularly true within the aesthetic areas of art, music, theatre, dance, and creative writing. In each of this, the individual is given the opportunity to make a unique expressive statement that is his alone. Within recreation, there need be no such limit, and the individual can be free to fully explore his latent creative abilities.

Physical Outcomes

In terms of physical outcomes, recreational activities obviously make an important contribution to the total well-being of the individual. Participating in sports, games, dance, or outdoor activities suited to one's age and general level of health and fitness is one of the surest ways to maintain an effectively functioning cardiovascular system and good muscular tone.

Emotional Outcomes

The ability to develop hobby interests or group ties, or to find emotional release through active sports or the expressive arts media, to find peace and relaxation in a natural setting, all of these are part of a well balanced regimen of living.

Intellectual Outcomes

One's recreational life may easily include attendance at the legitimate theatre or concerts, a great variety of reading, scientific pursuits, hobbies, exploration and travel, participation in adult courses and seminars, or similar pursuits. Provided that these are not work related, and have no other major extrinsic purposes, they are recreationally motivated.

Social Values of Recreation

From a societal point of view, when significant physical, emotional, social, and creative outcomes are derived from recreation for each individual participant, it enhances the quality of living in the society as a whole. When children, youth, adults and older citizens are all engaged in challenging, stimulating forms of leisure activity, or in helping to plan and organize community or agency programmes of recreation, this inevitably aids in creating a community in which desirable social values are stressed.

- It has frequently been pointed out that recreation is in itself no cure for juvenile delinquency, and to justify it on that sole basis would be fallacious. At the same time, however, it is widely recognized that attractive, challenging, and intelligently planned leisure time experiences, as an integrated part of a total community.
- Effectively supplement the work of the school, home, and temple in reducing delinquent behaviour.
- Realize the growing numbers of older persons find leisure a matter of deepest concern. If adequate recreational experiences are not provided, many older persons tend to sink into boredom, apathy, and physical and psychological degeneration. The community that makes concerted efforts to solve this problem, through the development and support of recreation programmes specifically geared to meet the needs of senior citizens, for happier and healthier place to live.

- Recreation offers the potential for knowing members of other racial, national, or religious groups better, for seeing them as individuals and not as stereotypes in short, for improving inter-group understanding and cooperation.

Economic Values of Recreation

In an economic sense, the importance of leisure and recreation for the nation comprises a major industry and absorbs a considerable portion of our productive energies. Each year, large new markets and fields of employment are being developed. What is not always so clearly understood is the extent to which recreation has positive economic value for the communities in which it exists. For every community, the extent to which it has come to grips with recreation needs may prove an important asset or serious liability. Nothing is more important to the physical and emotional health of the men and women of industry than proper recreation activities. So important is this considered that few modern companies would consider locating a new plant or facility in a community without first surveying its recreation possibilities.

Recreational Needs for Elderly

The aged in India is facing an unpleasant situation due to an increasingly industrialized and materialistic society and to a city that does not have enough space for its citizens. There are few open spaces earmarked for the elderly and their space within their homes is continually dwindling. Even as poor health catch up with them, they are faced with diminishing age finances, social isolation, loneliness, excessive free time and loss of family and friends. In fact, the 60+ citizens are the fastest growing age group in the country. Among the elderly itself, the growth rate of 80+ is the highest. Sheilu Srinivasan of the Dignity Foundation says that, by 2050, India will have the largest elderly population in the world. Yet, care for the aged is amongst the youngest of 'causes' in India. Children's rights and women's rights, though relatively new, have been around for decades; but 'rights of the aged' is a nascent concept. It is subsumed under the Ministry of Social Welfare and is ranked only after women and children.

Ageing is a time of multiple illness and general disability. Along with the changes in the biological compositions, lifestyle factors are also important for disorders and diseases in old age. Old age diseases are not always curable, implying a strain on financial as well as physical health infrastructure resources, both at the macro and micro levels. However, the feeling of well-being can still override actual physical discomforts if the surrounding environment is nurturing.

Support from the Community

There are institutions in Mumbai that seek to provide succour and recreation to the aged.

The three kinds of institutions that address different needs of senior citizens are:

1. Day care centres,
2. Residential old age homes, and
3. Associations of retired persons or of senior citizens.

It has been found that the services of 55 per cent of old age homes are free, 27 per cent charge varying rates for a senior citizen's stay, and 18 per cent have a regular fee structure. None of the three categories of institutions are evenly spread across the city. While 74 per cent of old age homes and the day care centres are within the city limits, 80 per cent of senior citizens' associations are in the western suburbs. A day care centre Family Welfare Agency (FWA), has launched recently a initiative to network all the organizations that deal with the elderly in an attempt to make their lives easier and enhance their accessibility to help. This initiative seeks to rope in the local civic wards, police stations, other public offices, voluntary organizations and volunteers in the interest of the aged. The idea of a day care centre for senior citizens is fast catching up. A few day care centres have come up in the city. Two such day care centres that seek to provide recreational, social and emotional support are Manav Seva Sangh and Family Welfare Agency. It offers varied indoor games like pool, table tennis, chess and carom; it also has medical facilities like services of a physiotherapist and holds sessions on techniques of alternative healing. It facilitates interaction between senior citizens and college students by inviting students to interact with the elderly. A full 24-hour helpline for senior citizens in distress is also on the anvil and the Sangh proposes to organize a volunteer service by other senior citizens, says social worker Vineeta Joshi. The helpline would offer medical advice, legal and social support, safety and security counselling, referral services, etc. The FWA also offers recreation like music, games, picnics and socio-cultural activities and counselling and legal services as well. Its day care units attract retired lower class pensioners.

Social Support Groups

Social Support provides recreational activities a small contribution as it assist with the cost of meals, transport and programme activities. Referrals may be made to the Social Support team leader or programme development officer. Social support groups consist of:

- Social groups for older people
- Arts, exercise and outdoor activities
- Social programmes for those living in supported residential services
- Career support groups and activities.

Older Adult Fitness and Health Activities

- Improve muscular and bone strength
- General well-being
- Relax muscles
- Provide an opportunity for fun
- Improve mobility and balance
- Improve joint flexibility

Suggestions for Recreational Activities

The following activities are recreational when performed during leisure, voluntarily, for the satisfaction inherent and for the socially accepted benefits they impart to the individual.

Arts and crafts: Activities, usually manual, such as drawing, modelling, painting, sculpting, sewing, photography, weaving and woodworking, which provide a creative outlet and expression.

Cultural activities: Activities such as arts and crafts, dance, drama, special events and sports that have special historical, ethnological or social significance for the participant. Examples are holiday ceremonies, pageants, and national celebrations. Cultural activities are often described as custom, tradition or folklore.

Dance: Activities which provide for rhythmic expression through patterned movements in a folk, social, modern and classical style.

Drama: Activities which provide opportunity for creative expression through storytelling, skits, plays, pageants and shows.

Entertainment: Activities of a passive nature such as television and radio or theatre or sports events which engage the attention in a satisfying manner.

Hobbies: Activities which are characterized by the participant's interest over a long period of time, for example, collecting antiques, coins and stamps, or cooking, gardening and home mechanics.

Mental and literary: Activities such as reading, discussion groups, card games, public speaking, game board activities and writing which provide intellectual outlet and creative expression.

Music: Activities such as listening to or participating in glee clubs, bands and concerts which provide expression through rhythm and melody.

Nature: Activities such as camping, hiking and nature study that involve being in using or interpreting the natural environment.

Social: Activities such as parties, picnics, banquets and club meetings engaged primarily for the satisfaction of social experience.

Special events: Organized activities that require special planning, for example, celebrations of special days and holidays, festivals and fairs.

Sports, games and athletics: Activities involving gross physical movement such as low organized, informal games, e.g. tag and relays; individual, dual and team sports usually requiring facilities and equipments, e.g., track and field meets.

Tourism: Activities such as outings and hostelling to sites of historical, cultural and natural interest that are characterized by travel away from one's home without remuneration.

Voluntary service: Activities such as being board member, group leader, team coach or instructor, those are inherently satisfying. They are performed voluntarily for the benefit of the community.

From the above suggestions, we can improve the mental health status of the people in our society such as elderly, women and children. These suggestions are implemented to all of them. It helps to build knowledge and rid of depression. One should follow and implement these given suggestions to improve their lifestyle and mental health.

Conclusion

Recreation and leisure service has a vital role to play in efforts to improve the lives of people living under adverse conditions. Recreation has a role in family, child and youth welfare; rural development; service to the aged, the ill, and other individuals in need of special attention. The emerging effort in recreation and leisure services is part of a larger effort in the nation through education, employment, health and social welfare.

Recreation Service

Organized help, aid or assistance which provides individuals with the opportunity to have the experience known as recreation, generally, local recreation service is characterized by the provision of financing, personnel and leadership, equipment, facilities, supplies and the organization of activities. The recreation programme is the combined result.

Recreation Personnel

Titles include, among others, the following: superintended of recreation (parks), recreation camp, centre, programme, recreation leader, extension specialist, playground or play leader, etc.

Recreation Facilities

Types include, among others, outdoor; game courts and fields; sports areas and facilities; structures such as band shells, outdoor theatres, swimming pools; equipment such as fireplaces, picnic facilities, gardens, parks, playgrounds, community centres, single use such as museums, libraries, theatres, restaurants and facilities in recreation buildings such as cardrooms, lounges and stages.

Recreational Activities

- To open sports clubs in rural and urban areas.
- To construct grounds/stadium to encourage sports and games especially among the youth.
- To start gymkhanas.
- To organize for training in sports/games both indoor and outdoor.
- To purchase sports material, awards, prizes, and financial aid to sport person.

- Organize films shows, dance, orchestras, etc.
- To plant tree under various projects and schemes.

References

Astin, D.R. (1982) *Therapeautic Recreation Process and Technique*. John Wiley and Sons, Canada.

Kleindienst, V.K. and A. Weston. (1978) *The Recreational Sports Programme*. Prentice Hall, London.

Kraus, R.G. (1964) *Recreation and the Schools*. The Macmillan Company, New York and Collier Macmillan Limited, London.

Murphy, J.E. (1954) *Recreational Cultural Activities in Social Education*. Indian Adult Education Association, New Delhi.

Nesbitt, J.A. and P.D. Brown. (1970) *Recreation and Leisure Service for the Disadvantaged*. Lea and Febiger, Philadelphia.

Webliography

http://phm-india.org/pdf/nha2/Women_Health.PDF.

http://www.merinews.com/catFull.jsp?articleID=129696

http://aja.co.in/services.html

http://mentalhealth.samhsa.gov/publications/allpubs/CA-0006/default.asp

http://www.mentalhealtharticles.net/depression/depression-in-children.html

8

Ageing Workforce in the German Labour Market

Review of Intervention Strategies Adopted by Prestigious German Organizations

MEETA AGARWAL AND VEENA GANDOTRA

The United States has identified global ageing as one of the top three socio-economic issues facing planet earth in the 21st century (other two are global warming and global terrorism). In the United States there are 18.4 million workers aged 55 or older—a figure representing the 13 per cent of the workforce. By 2015, this number is projected to grow to 31.9 million or approximately, one in every five employee (US General Accounting Office, 2003). Similarly, 41 per cent of the Canadian working population is expected to be between the ages of 45 and 64 by the year 2021 (Avery et al., 2007). In the United Kingdom, 30 per cent of the workers are over 50 per cent (Dixon, 2003). The impact of ageing population is higher in West German state, although it was on rise earlier in the eastern parts of Germany. Moreover, in urban areas like Munich relative increase of ageing population was minimal while in rural areas like Bavaria more than 60 per cent of population belong to 55 to 64 years (Kirpal and Kuhl, 2006). As a whole across, the European Union, the proportion of workers over 50 is expected to rise nearly 25 per cent over the next 15 years (Turning boomers into boomerangs, 2006).

The 'graying' of the working population is expected to affect the social policies of work organizations. Large numbers of workers have

Figure 1A *Forecasted Demographic Development of Different Age Groups*

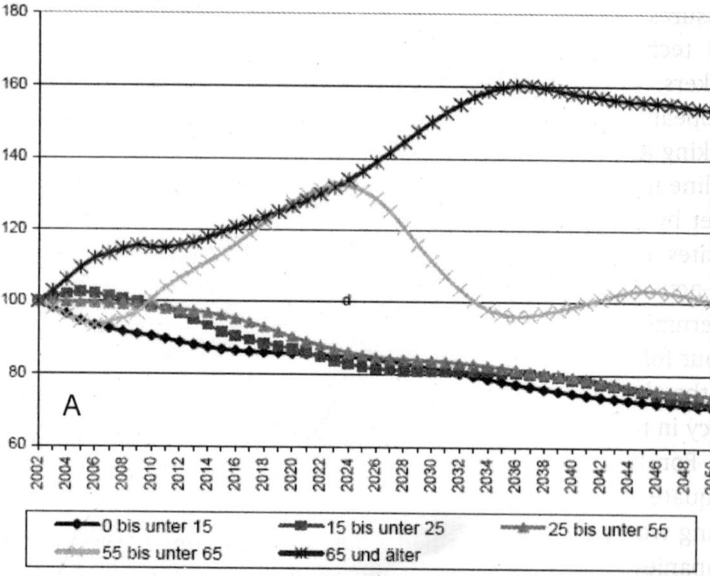

Figure 1B *Size of Youngest (15–24) and Oldest (55–64) Working Age Group for Germany*

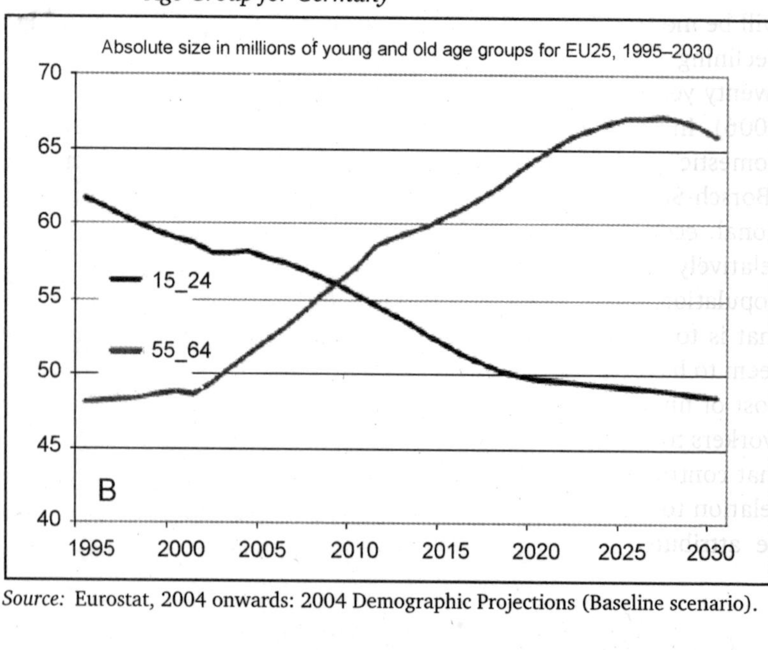

Source: Eurostat, 2004 onwards: 2004 Demographic Projections (Baseline scenario).

been forced to leave the labour market because the demands of work have become too high, resulting in inability to work. Increased time pressures, emotional stress from reorganizations or introduction of new technologies have been putting high demands on old aged workers. A much discussed demographic challenge faced by the European Union is not only the decline in the number of people of working age but also the strain on health and social security system. Decline in the relative size of economically active population will be offset by higher capital intensity (Borsch-Supan, 2003, 2004). This debates focus on the ratio between the economically active and non-active population. In their capacity as macro level actors, the government and social partners are aware of the need to raise the labour force participation of the older workers (Remery et al., 2003) but they lack concrete ideas and the instruments needed to flash out policy in this area.

For European countries, including Germany, how to provide adequate skills and lifelong learning environments for managing ageing workforce have become major *concern* for policy makers and companies during the past two decades (Illmarinen, 2005). Researches also reflect that Germany will encounter a severe mismatch of skills in the near future which for some areas and sectors will be more significant. The already existing mismatch is Germany's declining investment in human capitals formation during the past twenty years of education and training particulars (Kirpal and Kuhl, 2006). In order to compensate the impact of population ageing on domestic production, labour productivity will need to increased (Borsch-Supan, 2003). Demographic change may also alter international economic relations. Capital will flow from countries of relatively older population to countries of relatively young population where the rate of return is high. Despite the 'Gray' wave that is to inundate the labour market, individual employers do not seem to have a sense of urgency to act on this development. A whole host of financial measures are being implemented to encourage the workers to withdraw from labour force; there are very few incentives that contribute to alter the skills and knowledge of older workers in relation to innovative technologies. The lack of such measures may be attributed to the fact that employers tend to associate older workers primarily with low productivity, in particular given their higher, age related wage costs (Remery et al., 2003).

Review of Intervention Strategies Adopted by Various Organizations

Since most decisions on how to deal with an ageing workforce will have to be taken within individual organizations or at least be implemented within these organizations, therefore to look into the roles played by the different employers is important. Employers from Asia Pacific—most developed countries believe that the most important actions necessary to adapt to an ageing workforce are enhanced training and development together with later retirement (Ageing Workforce, 2006). The Adecco Institute surveyed companies across Europe to cope up with the demographic crunch, i.e., the challenge of an ageing workforce. Five factors were used to measures the company's fitness: career management, lifelong learning, knowledge management, health management and diversity management. Companies were graded on a scale of 100 to 400 points. The findings showed that UK and Germany were most prepared for an ageing workforce with average score of 186 compared to 182 in Italy, 180 in Spain and 174 in France. However, none of the five major European Union economies reaches a satisfactory Demographic Fitness Index (DFX). The goal of DFX is to raise the companies' awareness for demographic challenges which includes better analysis of age structure, the growing openness towards older employees and a strong commitment to improved education and trainings (www.clearlybusiness.com). Frerichs and Sporket (2007) reported that information and awareness campaigns, special labour market policies for older workers such as wage subsidies and funds for vocational trainings, raising age limits for different pensions and other initiatives are being taken by the Federal Government to increase the labour market participation of older workers.

Case Studies of Companies in Germany

European Foundation for the Improvement of Living and Working Conditions (www.eurofound.europa.eu) reported case studies of various companies situated in Germany. Some of them are summarized below:

Company	*Background*	*Percentage of Ageing Workforce*	*Intervention Strategies*
Wilkhahn	Makes top quality seats and tables for meeting and conference rooms, and offices.	Average age of employees is above 43 years. 13% older than 55 years.	Health promotion measures and skills training financed by the state of Lower Saxony and the European Union.
KSB Corporation	Leading manufacturer of pumps and valves for private and industrial applications worldwide.	Average age of employees 42 years. 33% are over 50 years of age.	Project with the support of the Rhineland-Palatinate's Ministry of Labour, Social Affairs and Family; Employee survey; Two workshops with older employees; Age-based workplaces; Specific trainings; Release from night shifts; Flexible working times; Mentor models for transferring expertise and easing older employees' workloads; Health checks; Preparation for retirement.
The Free Hanseatic City of Bremen	A combined state and local government administration	Average age of employees 42 years. 27.4% of prison officers are over 50 years old.	'Innovation to safeguard the future'.
Volkswagen Commercial Vehicles	The largest auto manufacturer in Europe.	The average age of production workers is 39.5 years.	Rotating and extending tasks; 'Cascade Model'—prevention, integration, integration department and special assembly—encompass all the measures required to maintain and restore workers employability and productivity; working life biographies.
Bosch Group	Manufacturer of innovative high-grade automotive and industrial technology, consumer goods.		Qualifications programme in cooperation with the Magdeburg employment office, Otto-von-Guericke University, Magdeburg, the Elop Institute in Magdeburg and Dresden and the TÜV Akademie to offer senior engineers re-enter in the labour market.

Cont'd...

Cont'd...

Rowenta Werke GmbH	Manufacturer of small household appliances, cast iron manufacturer.	More than 46% of employees are aged over 45 years.	Health management, health circles, employee's survey, job rotation, part time work (five hour shift).
Loewe AG	Listed company in the electrical industry.	More than 25% of employees are aged over 50 years	Project 67'-'Mastering the future with experience'. Labour market initiative 'Perspective 50 plus' -Four action areas: (a) management development and competence management, (b) job rotation in final assembly, (c) job enrichment in manual assembly and realignment of workplace and (d) health promotion.
Munich-base d BMW Group	Manufactures of automobiles and motorcycles	Above the age of 50 years totaled about 15%.	'Today for tomorrow' health management, qualifications, work environment, retirement models and change management.
OHG Netto Supermarkt GmbH	Subsidiary of a Danish supermarket chain	Total workforce of 3,000 employees in Germany, including 200 apprentices	'45+ supermarket' healthy age mix.
SICK AG	Manufacturers of sensors and sensor solutions.	About 68% of the employees aged between 30 and 49 years. The average age is under 40 years.	Life course-oriented personnel development, mixed-age project teams, diversification at work-job rotation, health promoting issues: communications training, training of executives, qualification of group work, stress management training, time management training, health checks, health counselling and health days and working group to encourage sports activities.

Cont'd...

Cont'd...

Sozial-Holding der Stadt Mönchengladbach GmbH	Coordinates community care services for the elderly and other care services.	Around 25% of its employees are over 50 years of age	health management programme-to reduce the health risks associated with the workplace, introducing the 'daily apple' as a symbol for Health-conscious behaviour and as a sign of the company's willingness to support its employees, 'health circles' vocational training on gerontology and work organization including correct lifting and carrying techniques. Employee suggestion system and annual employee appraisal system for information exchange and feedback about the employee's positive and negative developments. promoting the motto, 'we are older than 50—so what?'
Fahrion Engineering GmbH & Co KG	Medium-sized engineering company	42% of all employees are over 50	Mixed-age teams career and life options at diff. age-36+: annual career-management talks, 55+: situation talks with the family, 60+: dual project management (an older and a younger employee work together to transfer knowledge and to relieve the older worker of responsibilities before retirement), 62+: extending the retirement age through partial retirement.
Die Continentale	Health insurance company	21% of the employees are aged over 50 years.	European project 'active@work'—alternative work arrangements, mixed-age workforces; HR policy in 7 areas: personnel recruitment, knowledge preservation, maintaining productivity levels, developing innovativeness, organizational culture, sales development and managing staff turnovers

Research Gap

Despite the various recommendations and implications that we found from different case studies and researches, there is still a significant research gap in terms of how management should solve the problem of the ageing workforce both in terms of older workers needs and organizational benefits. There exist contradictions between official statements and beliefs of the companies' employers association and the actual treatment of older workers in the company. In Germany, companies are less interested in providing the training to older workforce. Kirpal and Kuhl (2006) reported that only 1 per cent of companies are offering training that is particularly oriented towards the needs of the older workers. Differences were also observed based on large/small company's set-up. The large companies which rely on innovative technologies and are profit oriented are more likely to invest in training of their employee than the medium and smaller ones. Moreover, company's human resource development strategies are targeted towards employees of below 45 years of age (Streb et al., 2008). Employee's competence and career development needs are not systematically and strategically supported by the employers. Lifelong learning policies and implementation strategies at European level aims self-initiatives and self-directed learning. But older workers are not familiar with such type of learning. Further, many initiatives like information and awareness campaigns, special labour market policies for older workers like wage subsidies and funds for vocational trainings, raising age limits for different pensions and other initiatives are being taken by Federal Government, yet there is no public policy for older workers. Trade unions have not succeeded in negotiating internal company's measures to retain older workers by increasing training provisions for them. There is still need to develop an effective research tool for combating the problem of ageing workforce in a more effective manner. How older workers will be supported at macro level and policies and behaviours at micro level are to be studied. Data base of case studies offers an up-to-date resource of ideas, initiatives and incentives to respond to demands for better age management at workplace. But still there is need for increasing the level of awareness and commitment and stimulating change in all organizations. Changes in early exit and retirement policies of companies need to be addressed.

References

Ageing Workforce Report. (2006) Watsonwyatt.com

Avery, D.R., P.F. McKay and D.C. Wilson. (2007) *Journal of Applied Psychology*, Vol. 92, No. 6, pp. 1542–1556.

Borsch-Supan, A. (2003) "Labour Market Effects of Population Ageing". *Journal of Labour*, Vol. 17, pp. 5–44.

Borsch-Supan, A. (2004) Global Ageing: Issues, Answers, More Questions. University of Michigan Retirement Research Centre, Research Paper No. WP–2004–084.

Dixon, S. (2003) "Implications of Population Ageing for the Labour Market". *Labour Market Trends*, National Statistics Office, London, Vol. 111, No. 2, pp. 67–76.

European Foundation for the Improvement of Living and Working Conditions. http://www.eurofound.europa.eu

Frerichs, F. and M. Sporket. (2007) Employment and Labour Market Policies for an Ageing Workforce Initiatives at the Working Place. Overview Report, Germany.

Illmarinen, J. (2005) *Towards a Longer Worklife: Ageing and the Quality of Worklife in the European Union*. Finnish Institute of Occupational Health, Helsinki.

Kirpal, S. and A. Kuhl. (2006) Sustaining Older Workers' Competence: Case Study Germany. Paper presented in European Conference on Educational Research (ECER, 2006), Geneva, September 13–16.

Remery, C., K. Henkens, J. Schippers and P. Ekamper. (2003) "Managing an Ageing Workforce and a Tight Labour Market: Views held by Dutch Employers". *Population Research and Policy Reviews*, Vol. 22, pp. 21–40.

Streb, C.K., S.C. Voelpel and M. Leibold. (2008) "Managing the Ageing Workforce: Status Quo and Implications for the Advancement of Theory and Practice". *European Management Journal*, Vol. 26, pp. 1–10.

Turning boomers into boomerangs. (2006) *The Economist Print Edition*. https://www.azdes.gov/aaa/programmes/owp/docs/The%20Economist%202-16-06.

United States General Accounting Office. (2003) Older Workers: Policies of Other Nations to Increase Labour Force Participation. Washington DC.

9

Clothing for Third Age Women

PARUL DAVE AND VANDANA R. CHAUHAN

Over the last few decades, traditional Indian society has undergone radical changes. Older people once enjoyed a sense of authority, respect and honour. They were responsible for decision-making and were revered by all members of the family. All this has changed with the new generation due to modernization, urbanization and especially rise in nuclear families. The elderly are thereby forced to some extent to stay away from the son's family.

Ageing is a universal process and no individual can escape it. It has been defined by Maynard-Smith (1962) as "the process which renders individuals more susceptible as and when they grow order, to various factors intrinsic or extrinsic, which may cause death", recognizing that death may arise from a decline in the individual organism's ability to maintain its intrinsic function in the face of psychological stress from an extrinsic source such as 'accidents' or 'disease' (Bond et al., 1999).

Ageing has been defined as, "A collective term for all those progressive deteriorating changes that occur in life with an increase in age" (Gowli et al., 2003). The ageing process is the culmination of the psychological, social and biological factors which results in decline or deterioration. It is not a homogenous experience that affects every individual within the same society in the same manner.

The ageing process varies within and amongst cultures. Becoming old results in social, biological, psychological and cultural change, which ultimately results in relinquishing the roles played till now to someone else, displacement from the position of power and an increase in dependency on the family and society.

In traditional Indian family and society, age had value in itself, regardless of religion or caste. The older persons were venerated because they were repositories of wisdom, experience, custom and property rights. Their contribution in the field of education, socialization, social control, transmission of cultural values and heritage to the future generation cannot be underestimated.

India is witnessing a silent demographic revolution due to steady growth of its older population. This demographic marvel is accompanied by the diverse problems faced by the elderly related to health, housing, income and an array of socio-psychological issues especially by the ageing women.

Further, there is a considerable diversity amongst various age groups of the elderly, that is young-old or old-old. This difference is marked in the area of health and well-being. Similarly, gender, social status and marital status determine the quality of life in later years. It becomes necessary to differentiate between old men and women as gender is a powerful factor affecting quality of life at all stages of life.

Women in the developing world experience low social status, poor reproductive heath care, economic dependence, malnutrition and domestic violence, which affect their well-being adversely. Over the life cycle such disadvantages accumulate leaving older women in a venerable condition. They are looked down first as women and secondly as aged women. Hence, the women above 60 years constitute a special concern group in the general population.

The United Nations projects that by the year 2025, there will be 604 million women over the age 60 in the world population. Seventy per cent of these will be in the Third World countries. Especially, with reference to India, such global view of 'gender ageing' reveals the situation of older Indian women as highly vulnerable due to decreasing physical capacity and mobility, increasing financial and psychological dependence, lack of availability of support network and ignorance about their rights.

Objectives

Clothing, an integral part of the human life, satisfies functional, social and aesthetic needs of all people of all ages. The expanded life span of the elderly has major implication on the clothing pattern and style maintained by them. With decrease in physical strength, it is necessary to design clothes which are easy to put on or take off and easy to care. Clothing also plays in important part in rendering a sense of well-being, socially and acceptance in a society. Women who attend fewer organizations stated that lack of appropriate attire affected their feeling of ease in the social gathering and hence they refused invitations. Thus, wardrobe size and type, influence the social life.

The stereotypical image implies that older people do not care about their appearance. Hurlock (1981) reported that interest in clothes to some extent depends on how socially active the elderly are, partly on economic status and partly on how willing they are to accept the fact that they are growing old and must adjust to it (Goyal, 2000). Some people continue to wear styles they wore earlier and refuse to dress according to the current fashion. But, on the other hand, there are fashion-conscious elderly as well, who dress according to the existing trends. These tendencies show a diverse view of either clinging to the youth or rebelling against old age and trying to convince others and themselves that they are younger than reality.

Limited income forces many older people from having much interest in their clothes and appearances as they might otherwise have. Sometimes physical changes that occur in the body with advancing age, limits the choices available to them.

Clothing should be such that it is neat, clean, fits well and boosts the morale. It should make older people feel better about themselves, irrespective of age and physical limitations. It is important that older person's garments must be designed with relation to their health problems, physical decline, kind of activity performed as well as seasonal variation. Thus, it should serve the purpose of comfort, convenience and should be appropriate to suite the climatic conditions.

Indian national data on clothing requirements and clothing preferences of the older persons is not available. The present project tries to fill this lacunae and would help to understand the clothing requirements of elderly women.

Goals

- To understand the clothing practices, needs and preferences of older women and their socio-cultural and socio-economic background.

- To identify the need for specially designed clothes considering health status (physical ailments), seasonal changes and comfort for older women.

Methodology

The present study was conducted by Prof. Parul Dave (Project Coordinator), Women's Studies Research Centre, The M.S. University of Baroda, Vadodara in March 2005.

Vandana R. Chauhan was on the research team as investigator from the field of clothing and textiles.

This research paper deals with the clothing practices, needs and preferences of older women. It also encompasses the need for special designed clothes considering health status, seasonal changes and comfort for older women.

The present study was descriptive and exploratory in nature and was conducted in the urban settings of Vadodara city having a population of more than 13 lakh, of which 6.19 per cent make up people above 60 years of age, with almost an equal number of males and females.

A semi-structural interview schedule and a questionnaire to assess the quality of life of older women was prepared.

The tools were prepared in English and then translated into Gujarati for better comprehension by the respondents and ease in communication. Content validity was done. Pilot study was carried out. All necessary changes were made and the questionnaire was finalized. It was then executed.

Sample Selection

A stratified sample was selected using a purposive criteria, from the population of elderly women residing in Vadodara city. The criteria for sample selection are as follows:

Age: Older women, who were at least 60 years of age or above, were selected. The years were divided into categories of young-old and old-old women. The young-old group represented women in the age range of 60–75 years whereas the old-old group included women above the age of 75+ years.

Living arrangements: Besides age, living arrangement is an important variable determining the quality of life of older women. Thus, the sample included women from both age groups who were:

- Living alone
- Living with spouse
- Living with family

Socio-economic Status

An effort was made to identify the sample from the middle and upper-middle class, to maintain uniformity. The reason for selecting middle and upper-middle income groups was that these stratas are expected to be relatively educated and may be either a part of paid labour market or might be playing a role in decision-making in the household.

Procedure

Various organizations working with the older persons in Vadodara were contacted, to identify a sample fulfilling the above-mentioned criteria. After primary identification and contacts with some respondents, the snowball technique was used to identify other respondents.

The total sample size for the study was 180 respondents. This was further divided into two age groups of young-old and old-old women, consisting of 75 elderly women each. Further division into groups of 25 women was made on the basis of kind of living arrangement. Figure 1 represents the sample design.

Figure 1 *Sample Design*

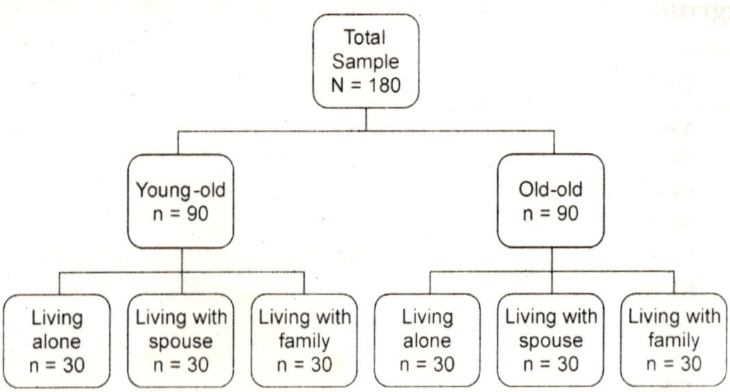

Development of Tool

A semi-structured interview schedule and a questionnaire to assess the quality of life of older women were prepared with inputs from the core team members. Background information of the respondents was also obtained.

The tools were prepared in English and then translated into Gujarati for better comprehension by the respondents and ease in communication. The content validity of the tools with their sub-sections, was established through feedback from core team members.

Pilot Study

The tool was pilot tested on a sample of 18 respondents selected for the purpose. These respondents met all the criteria of sample selection but were not a part of the main study. Pilot study yielded the following feedback.

- An estimate of time taken for administration of the tool
- Extent of suitability and comprehension of questions by the respondents.

The results of the pilot test helped to simplify the language and reduce the time taken for its administration.

Data Analysis

Bivariate tables with frequencies and percentages were prepared for the data pertaining to clothing and textiles.

Results, Discussion and Conclusions

Background Information

	Characteristics	*Frequency (N=180)*	*%*
(A)	**Age Distribution**		
	60–64	40	22.2
	65–69	24	13.3
	70–74	26	14.4
	75–80	56	31.2
	81–84	22	12.2
	> 85	12	6.7
		180	100.00
(B)	**Education**		
	Primary	65	36.1
	Metric (10th pass)	28	15.6

Cont'd..

Cont'd...

	High school (12th pass)	12	6.7
	Graduate	38	21.1
	Post-graduate	32	17.8
	illiterate	5	2.7
		180	100.00
(C)	**Religion**		
	Hindu	160	88.9
	Christian	4	2.2
	Muslim	7	3.8
	Punjabi	2	1.1
	Zarastrian/Parsi	3	1.7
	Jain	3	1.7
	Sikh	1	0.6
		180	100.00
(D)	**Mother Tongue**		
	Gujarati	139	77.2
	Marathi	23	13.3
	Malayalam	3	1.7
	Tamil	6	3.3
	Hindi	7	3.8
	Punjabi	1	1.6
		180	100.00
(E)	**Marital Status**		
	Unmarried	9	5.0
	Married	92	51.1
	Widowed	77	42.8
	Divorced/Separated	2	1.1
		180	100.00
(F)	**Type of Family**		
	Nuclear	124	69.1
	Joint	54	30.1
	NA*	2	1.1
		180	100.00

NA* = No family members are living.

The background information of respondents comprised of the following characteristics:

(a) Age Group
(b) Education
(c) Religion
(d) Mother Tongue

(e) Martial Status

(f) Type of Family

- The data collected revealed 31.2 per cent of the respondents belonged to the age group of 75–80 years. Also 22.2 per cent belonged to the group of 60–64 years.
- The education of 36.1 per cent of elderly women was upto primary and 21.1 per cent respondents were graduate. Only 2.7 per cent of them were illiterate.
- A majority (88.9%) of the respondents followed Hindu religion. The other religions followed were Christianity (2.2%), Muslim (3.8%), Sikh (1.6%), Parsi (1.7%) and Jainism (1.7%).
- With respect to mother tongue again a majority (77.2%) of the respondent spoke Gujarati whereas 13.3 per cent adopted Marathi. The other languages were Malayalam (1.7%), Tamil (3.3%), Hindi (3.8%) and Punjabi (1.6%).
- As far as martial status was concerned a little more than half (51.1%) of the respondents were married. Due to elderly age 42.8% per cent of the respondents were widowed.
- Again a majority (69.1%) of the respondents had a nuclear family and 30.1% per cent had a joint family.

Daily Activity Schedule

A day in the life of women of third age:

Timings	*Activities*
6:00 am to 9:00 am	Rise and do morning ablutions. Prayers at home of at the temple walk/exercise. Breakfast. Reading newspaper.
9:00 am to 11:00 am	Preparing lunch. Household chores like cleaning, dusting, cutting vegetables, washing light clothes and supervising hired help.
12 noon to 2:00 pm	Lunch with family. Cleaning kitchen
2:00 pm to 4:00 pm	Rest time and sleep. Watch television
4:00 pm to 5:00 pm	Tea. Indulge in chit-chat with family. Light chores like folding clothes, arranging washed utensils.
5:00 pm to 8:00 pm	Leisure time. Watching television. Chatting with neighbours, friends. Social visits. Spending time with grandchildren. Going to temple or for a walk. Help or prepare dinners.
8:00 pm to 10:00 pm	Dinner time. Watch television. Interact with family
10:00 pm to 12:00 midnight	Sleep

The schedule shows that a reasonable amount of time was spent in household activities by the respondents.

Religious activities were carried out by the elderly women throughout the day. These activities comprised of puja or prayers, reciting 'mantras' or god's name using beads, watching religious programmes on television in the morning, reading religious books in the afternoon and in the evening most of the respondents went to the temple.

Sundays and other public holiday were mostly same for the respondents unless if they had guests at their place or they were out of station.

Clothes have been the fascination to enhance person's appearance as well as to boost morale, regardless of age. It satisfies functional, social and aesthetic need of people of all ages. Thus clothes not only serve the utilitarian purpose of covering the body but also add beauty and elegance to an individual's personality. Apart from this, it has a social and psychological impact.

The expanded life span due to advances in medical sciences has brought many new problems relating old age, some of which have implication for clothing. However, for this particular population clothing needs have by and large been left unrecognized, though clothes have a tremendous psychological and therapeutic effect. Clothing needs of the older persons gained special attention in American studies during the early 20th century and the need for designed clothes for older population was also recognized.

The present section on results and analysis comprises of:

- Wardrobe type and size
- Clothing preferences
- Maintenance of garments
- Shopping practices
- Factors influencing clothing pattern

Saree

As seen in Table 1, in both the groups it was seen that more number of respondents have sarees less than or equal to 30 (in number).

- In the young group, varied responses are seen. 32.2 per cent respondents have sarees numbering 30, 25.6 per cent have sarees between 31 and 60, 10 per cent have 61–90 sarees, while 21.1 per cent have sarees more than 90.

Table 1 *Wardrobe Type and Size*

Age Group		*Young-Old*							
Total No.	*Garments Living Arrangements*	*A*	*B*	*C*	*D*	*E*	*F*	*G*	*H*
< 30	LA	46.60	53.30	60.00	13.30	.000	3.30	16.70	13.30
	LS	16.70	23.40	76.70	30.00	10.00	6.70	56.60	3.30
	LF	33.30	33.30	70.00	10.00	3.30	0.00	43.30	0.00
	Total	32.2	36.67	68.9	17.77	4.43	3.33	38.77	5.53
31–60	LA	13.40	13.40	6.60	0.00	0.00	0.00	0.00	0.00
	LS	23.30	30.00	13.30	0.00	0.00	0.00	0.00	0.00
	LF	40.00	46.70	13.30	6.70	0.00	0.00	0.00	0.00
	Total	25.57	30.03	11.07	2.23	0.00	0.00	—	—
61–90	LA	13.30	6.70	6.70	0.00	0.00	0.00	0.00	0.00
	LS	23.40	16.60	0.00	0.00	0.00	0.00	0.00	0.00
	LF	6.60	0.00	3.30	0.00	0.00	0.00	0.00	0.00
	Total	14.43	7.77	3.33	—	—	—	—	—
> 90	LA	10.00	8.90	6.70	0.00	0.00	0.00	0.00	0.00
	LS	33.30	26.70	6.70	0.00	0.00	0.00	0.00	0.00
	LF	20.00	16.70	6.70	3.30	0.00	0.00	0.00	0.00
	Total	21.1	17.43	6.7	1.1	—	—	—	—
NA	LA								
	LS								
	LF								
	Total	6.6	7.8	10.0	78.9	95.6	96.7	60.0	94.4
Age Group		*Old-Old*							
Total No.	*Garments Living Arrangements*	*A*	*B*	*C*	*D*	*E*	*F*	*G*	*H*
< 30	LA	53.30	6.00	63.40	6.60	0.00	0.00	13.30	0.00
	LS	70.00	70.00	76.70	16.60	0.00	0.00	23.30	6.70
	LF	83.30	93.30	93.40	0.00	3.30	0.00	13.30	3.30
	Total	68.87	74.43	77.83	7.73	1.1	0	16.63	3.33
31–60	LA	16.70	13.30	10.00	0.00	0.00	0.00	0.00	0.00
	LS	20.00	20.00	16.60	0.00	0.00	0.00	0.00	0.00
	LF	13.30	3.30	3.30	0.00	0.00	0.00	0.00	0.00

Cont'd...

Cont'd...

	Total	16.67	12.2	9.97	0	0	0	0	0
61–90	LA	6.60	3.30	3.30	0.00	0.00	0.00	0.00	0.00
	LS	0.00	0.00	0.00	0.00	0.00	0.00	0.00	0.00
	LF	3.30	3.30	3.30	0.00	0.00	0.00	0.00	0.00
	Total	3.3	2.2	2.2	0	0	0	0	0
> 90	LA	10.00	10.00	10.00	0.00	0.00	0.00	0.00	0.00
	LS	6.60	6.70	3.30	0.00	0.00	0.00	0.00	0.00
	LF	0.00	0.00	0.00	0.00	0.00	0.00	0.00	0.00
	Total	5.53	5.57	4.43	0	0	0	0	0
NA	LA								
	LS								
	LF								
	Total	5.6	5.6	5.6	92.2	98.9	100.0	82.2	

Note: LA—Living alone; LS—Living with Spouse; LF—Living with family; YO—Young-old; OO—Old-old; NA—Not available

A: Saree, B: Saree-Blouse, C: Saree-Petticoat, D: Salwar-Kameez, E: Dress, F: Trouser Top, G: Gown, H: Any other.

- In the group where sarees number is 30, more respondents are seen in the living alone group, followed by living with family. In the group where saree numbered 31–60, more respondents living with family group followed by 23.3 per cent and after the 31–60 group, all respondents who live with spouse are more as compared to the other two living arrangement.

In the old group, maximum number of respondents have sarees 30, 68.9 per cent followed by 16.6 per cent respondents who have saree number 31–60, 3.3 per cent have 61–90 number of saree's, while 5.5 per cent have sarees more than 90 in number. No distinguishing features, about living arrangement could be seen.

Saree-Blouse

A pattern similar to saree is observed, where maximum respondents have saree-blouse (SB)30.

- In young group, varied response was seen as 36.6 per cent have SB less or equal to 30 in number, 30.03 per cent have SB 31–60 in number, 7.7 per cent respondents have 61–90 number of SB, while 17.4 per cent respondents have more than 90 SB. In the group where SB number is 30, respondents who live alone are more (53.3%), followed by respondents living with family. In group where SB number is 31–60, respondents living with family are more (46.7%), followed by respondents living with spouse. In groups 61–90 number and >90 number of SB, respondents living with spouse are more.

- In the older group maximum number of respondents have SB number 30 (74.43%). 31–60 number of SB are seen in 12.2 per cent respondents, 61–90 number of SB seen in 2.2 per cent respondents, while > 90 are seen in 5.53 per cent respondents.

Saree-Petticoat

Similar pattern to saree and saree-blouse was seen, where more number of respondents have saree-petticoat (SP)<30.

- In younger group, maximum number of respondents have SP 30 in number (68.9%), where the number of respondents living with the spouse was 76.7 per cent which was more, followed by living with family.
- 11.06 per cent respondents have SP 31–60 in number, where equal number of respondents were therein respondents who lived with family and respondents who lived with spouse.
- 3.3 per cent respondents have SP 61–90 in number, where more respondents are living alone and no respondents living with spouse have responded. 6.7 per cent respondents have SP > 90 in number, where equal number of respondents are present in all three groups.
- In older group, maximum number of respondents had SP 30 in number (77.8%), out of which 93 per cent respondents were living with family, followed by 76.7 per cent respondents living with spouse. 9.96 per cent respondents had SP 31–60 in number, in which 16.6 per cent respondents were living with spouse and 10 per cent respondents were living alone.
- 2.2 per cent respondents had SP 61–90 in number, where equal number of respondents were there who were living alone and living with family. >90 in number were seen in 4.43 per cent respondents, where 10 per cent respondents lived alone and 3.3 per cent lived with family.

Salwar-Kameez

- A total of 17.7 per cent respondents in YO group were maximum and had salwar-kameez, 30 in number, in which 30 per cent respondents lived with spouse, 13.3 per cent respondents lived alone and 10 per cent respondents lived with family. 2.2 per cent respondents have salwar-kameez 31–60 in number, in which 6.7 per cent respondents lived with family. 3.3 per cent respondents lived with family have salwar-kameez >90 number.

- In the older group, 7.73 per cent respondents have salwar-kameez 30 in number, in which 16.6 per cent live with family and 6.6 per cent live alone.

Dress

Dress is seen in only 4.43 per cent respondents in YO group and 1.1 per cent respondents in OO group, which had dress number 30.

In YO group, 10 per cent respondents living with spouse and 3.3 per cent respondents living with family have 30 dress. In OO group, 3.3 per cent respondents who lived with family have dress number as 30.

Trouser and Top

Trouser and top is seen in 3.3 per cent respondents in YO group only, in which 6.7 per cent respondents lived with spouse and 3.3 per cent respondents, lived alone.

Gown

38.8 per cent respondents, who wore gown, had it in 30 number, in YO group, in which 56.6 per cent respondents lived with spouse, 43.3 per cent lived with family and 16.7 per cent lived alone. 16.63 per cent respondents have gown 30 in number in OO group, in which 23.3 per cent respondents lived with spouse and 13.3 per cent respondents were there who were living alone and living with family respectively.

Number of Garments: Maximum number of respondents in both the groups have said they have adequate number of garments.

- 3.3 per cent respondents in the YO group, who live alone and 6.7 per cent respondents in the OO, who live with spouse have said that the number of garments they possess at present is inadequate.
- The respondents in the YO group who lived with spouse, said that the "I wear what is available". The respondents in OO group did not respond.

- As to number of garments required more no response was obtained.

Table 2 *Daily Pattern of Wearing Clothes*

Age Group			*Young-Old*							
Pattern		*Garments Living Arrange-ments*	*A*	*B*	*C*	*D*	*E*	*F*	*NA*	*NR*
Daily Wear	Day wear	LA	83.3	10.0	—	—	3.3	10.0	3.3	—
		LS	86.7	26.7	3.3	3.3	13.3	3.3	—	—
		LF	83.3	16.7	3.3	3.3	6.7	—	—	—
		Total	84.4	17.8	2.2	2.2	7.8	4.4	1.1	—
	Night wear	LA	70.0	—	3.3	—	26.7	10.0	—	—
		LS	46.7	6.7	—	—	60.0	3.3	—	—
		LF	40.0	6.7	—	—	53.3	—	—	—
		Total	52.2	4.4	1.1	—	46.7	4.4	—	—
Occasions	Festivals	LA	86.7	—	—	—	3.3	10.0	—	—
		LS	93.3	6.7	3.3	—	—	3.3	—	—
		LF	96.7	3.3	—	—	—	—	—	—
		Total	92.2	3.3	1.1	—	1.1	4.4	—	—
	Meeting friends and relatives	LA	83.3	3.3	—	—	—	10.0	—	3.3
		LS	86.7	20.0	6.7	3.3	—	3.3	—	3.3
		LF	86.7	3.3	—	—	—	—	6.7	3.3
		Total	85.6	8.9	2.2	1.1	—	4.4	2.2	3.3
Exercise	Morning walk	LA	26.7	6.7	—	3.3	3.3	—	—	60.0
		LS	53.3	20.0	—	6.7	—	—	—	30.0
		LF	43.3	10.0	—	6.7	3.3	—	6.7	33.3
		Total	41.1	12.2	—	5.6	2.2	—	2.2	41.1
	Evening walk	LA	23.3	—	—	3.3	—	—	—	73.3
		LS	56.7	23.3	—	—	—	—	6.7	20.0
		LF	46.7	10.0	—	3.3	3.3	—	13.3	26.7
		Total	42.2	11.1	—	2.2	1.1	—	6.7	40.0

Cont'd...

Cont'd...

Age Group			*Old-Old*							
Pattern	*Garments*	*Living Arrange-ments*	*A*	*B*	*C*	*D*	*E*	*F*	*NA*	*NR*
Daily Wear	Day Wear	LA	80.0	3.3	—	—	13.3	6.7	3.3	—
		LS	90.0	—						
	—	—	16.7	3.3	3.3	—				
		LF	96.7	3.3	—	—	6.7	—	—	—
		Total	88.9	2.2	—	—	12.2	3.3	2.2	—
	Night Wear	LA	63.3	6.7	—	—	23.3	6.7	3.3	—
		LS	60.0	—	—	—	40.0	3.3	6.7	—
		LF	76.7	—	—	—	23.3	3.3	—	—
		Total	66.7	2.2	—	—	28.9	4.4	3.3	—
Occasions	Festivals	LA	73.3	3.3	—	—	—	6.7	16.7	—
		LS	83.3	—	—	—	—	3.3	13.3	—
		LF	80.0	3.3	—	—	—	—	20.0	—
		Total	78.9	2.2	—	—	—	3.3	16.7	—
	Meeting friends and relatives	LA	66.7	6.7	—	—	—	6.7	23.3	—
		LS	80.0	10.0	—	—	—	3.3	10.0	—
		LF	80.0	—	—	—	—	—	20.0	—
		Total	75.6	5.6	—	—	—	3.3	17.8	—
Exercise	Morning walk	LA	13.3	—	—	—	3.3	—	83.3	—
		LS	6.7	—	—	—	—	—	93.3	—
		LF	20.0	—	—	—	—	—	80.0	—
		Total	13.3	—	—	—	1.1	—	85.6	—
	Evening walk	LA	13.3	—	—	—	3.3	—	83.3	—
		LS	10.0	—	—	—	—	—	90.0	—
		LF	20.0	—	—	—	—	—	80.0	—
		Total	14.4	—	—	—	1.1	—	84.4	—

Notes: A: Saree/Blouse/Petticoat, B: Salwar-kameez, C: Dress, D: Trouser and Top, E:Gown, F:Any other, NA: Not applicable, NR: No response.

Table shows multiple responses, All figures in percentages, NA: Respondents who do not do the activity.

Table 2 reveals that the pattern of wearing clothes for majority of the older people was saree/blouse/petticoat followed by dress and gown, in both the age groups. In the younger group, the respondents wearing gown for daily wear increases as compared to the older group.

Daily Wear

Clothes in Day Wear

Majority of respondents wore saree/petticoat/blouse during the day in the both the groups. A variety of pattern was observed in the younger group, where along with saree/blouse/petticoat, salwar kameez (17.8%), dress (2.2%), trouser and top (2.2%), gown (7.8) and other clothes (4.4%) were worn. In the older group this was not observed, where alongwith saree/blouse/petticoat, respondents wore salwar (2.2%), gown (12.2%) and other (3.3%) clothes.

- No major difference was observed in wearing of saree-blouse-petticoat in the younger group with respect to living arrangement, while in the older group more number of respondents who lived with family and lived with spouse wore saree-blouse-petticoat, as compared to those living alone.
- More number of respondents in the younger group (17.8%) wore salwar-kameez during the day, than older group. In the younger group, with respect to living arrangement respondents who live with spouse wear salwar-kameez more, as compared to living with family (16.7%) and living alone (10%). In the older group equal number of respondents in living alone and living with family wore salwar-kameez only.
- Dress was worn by 3.3 per cent respondents each in the category of living with spouse and living with family in the younger group, while in the older group it was not worn by anyone.
- *Trouser and Top*: Trouser and top was worn by 3.3 per cent respondents each in the category of living with spouse and living with family in the younger group, while in the older group it was not worn by anyone.
- *Gown:* Gown was worn by more number of respondents in the older group than younger group. In respondents who lived alone, more number of respondents in the older group wore gown (3.3% YO, 13.3% OO). Minor difference was found in respondents who lived with spouse, where more respondents were in the older group (16.7% OO, 13.3% YO). 6.7 per cent

respondents who lived with family in each group respectively wore gown during the day.

Night Wear

Majority of the respondents wore saree/blouse/petticoat during night in both the groups, followed by night-gown. A small percentage of respondents in the younger group wore salwar-kameez, dress and other clothes, while in the older group they wore salwar-kameez and other clothes.

- *Saree/Petticoat/Blouse:* More number of respondents in the older group wore saree/petticoat/blouse at night as compared to younger group (66.7% OO and 52.2% YO). In the younger group more respondents who lived alone (70%) wore saree at night, as compared to older group (63.3%). A difference is observed in respondents who lived with spouse, where more respondents are present in the older group (60%) as compared to younger group (46.7%). A large difference is observed in respondents who lived with family in both the groups, where more respondents are found in the older group (76.7%), than younger group (40%).
- *Salwar-kameez:* Salwar-kameez was worn more by the younger (4.4%) than older group (2.2%) at night. In the younger respondents an equal number of respondents in the living with spouse and living with family (6.7% each) wore salwar-kameez, while in the older group only respondents who lived alone wore it (6.7%).
- *Dress:* Dress was worn only by 3.3 per cent who lived alone in the younger group. No respondents in older group.
- *Gown:* Gown was worn more by the younger group (46.7%) than older group (28.9%). With respect to living arrangement respondents who lived with spouse are maximum in both the groups (60% YO and 40% OO). This is followed by respondents who lived with family (53.3%) and respondents who lived alone (26.7%) in the younger group, while an equal number of respondents (23.3% each) were present in the two groups in older group.

Occasions

Festivals

Most of the respondents wore saree/blouse/petticoat for festivals. This was more in the younger group (92.2%), than older group (78.9%).

- *Saree/blouse/petticoat:* In the younger group (92.2%), more number of respondents were found who lived with family (96.7%), followed by respondents who lived with spouse (93.3%) and lastly respondents who lived alone (86.7%). In the older group, more number of respondents were found in the category living with spouse (83.3%), followed by respondents living with family (80%) and lastly respondents who lived alone (73.3%).
- *Salwar-kameez:* Worn more by the younger group (3.3%) than older group (2.2%). 6.7 per cent respondents who lived with spouse and 3.3 per cent respondents who lived with family in the younger group wore salwar-kameez, while 3.3 per cent respondents each in the category of living alone and living with family wore it, during festivals.
- *Dress:* Dress was worn by 3.3 per cent respondents who lived with spouse in the younger group only.
- *Gown:* 3.3 per cent respondents who lived alone in the younger group only.

Meeting Friends and Relatives

Majority of the respondents wore saree/blouse/petticoat fro meeting friends and relatives. A small percentage wore salwar-kameez, dress and trouser and top.

- *Saree/blouse/petticoat:* More number of respondents in the younger group (85.6%) wore saree/blouse/petticoat as compared to older group (75.6%). An equal number of respondents who lived with spouse and lived with family wore saree in both the groups (86.7% in YO and 80% in OO), followed by more number of respondents who lived alone in younger group (83.3%), than older group (66.7%).
- *Salwar-kameez:* Worn more by the younger group (8.9%), than older group (5.6%). With respect to living arrangement, more respondents were those who lived with spouse (20%) YO and 10% OO), followed by 6.7 per cent respondents who lived alone in the older group, and an equal number of respondents in living alone and living with family (3.3%) are there in the younger group.
- *Dress:* Worn by 6.7 per cent respondents who lived with spouse in the younger group only.

- *Trouser-top:* 3.3 per cent respondents who lived with spouse in the younger group only.

Exercise

Morning Walk

Majority of the respondents wore saree/blouse/petticoat for morning walk, followed by salwar-kameez and trouser-top. More number of respondents were in the younger group, while it was seen that more number of respondents in older group do not go for morning walk.

- *Saree/Blouse/Petticoat:* There were more number of respondents in the younger group (41.1%) than older group (13.3%).
  - In the younger group, with respect to living arrangement more respondents were from the group who lived with spouse (53.3%) followed by respondents who lived with family (43.3%) and lastly respondents who lived alone (26.7%).
  - In the older group, more respondents were those who lived in family (20%), followed by respondents who lived alone (13.3%) and lastly respondents who lived with spouse (6.7%).
- *Salwar-kameez:* Worn by 12.2 per cent respondents in the younger group only, in which more respondents were from respondents who lived with spouse (20%), followed by respondents who lived with family (10%) and lastly respondents who lived alone (6.7%).
- *Trouser and Top:* 5.6 per cent respondents in the younger group wore trouser and top. In this equal number of respondents is those who lived with spouse and lived with family (6.7%) and followed by respondents who lived alone (3.3%).
- *Gown:* More number of respondents in the younger group (2.2%) wore 'gown' than older group (1.1%). In the younger group 3.3 per cent respondents in living alone and living with family respectively in the younger group wore gown, while 3.3 per cent respondents who lived alone in older group wore it.

Evening Walk

More number of respondents wore saree/blouse/petticoat, followed by salwar-kameez, trouser and top and gown, more response was seen in the younger group than older group.

Saree/Blouse/Petticoat: More number of respondents in the younger group wore saree/blouse/petticoat (42.2% YO), than older group (14.4%).

- In the younger group more number of respondents were found in the living with spouse (56.7%) category, followed by respondents who lived with family (46.7%) and lastly respondents who lived alone (23.3%).
- In the older group more numbers of respondents are in the living with family (20%), followed by respondents who lived alone (13.3%) and lastly respondents who lived with spouse (10%).

Salwar-kameez: Worn by 11.1 per cent respondents in the younger group only, in which more number of respondents were from respondents living with spouse (23.3%) followed by respondents living with family (10%).

Trouser and top: Worn by 3.3 per cent respondents each in the category of living alone and living with family.

Gown: Gown worn by equal number of respondents in both the groups, in which 3.3 per cent respondents who lived with family in the younger group and 3.3 per cent respondents who lived alone in the older group were present.

Any other: An equal number of respondents in both the groups respectively in the various patterns of wearing clothes during the day, wear other clothes like only blouse and petticoat, or a shirt, as they were unable to wear other garments due to disability. This was seen in 10 per cent respondents who lived alone and 3.3 per cent respondents who lived with spouse in the younger group, while 6.7 per cent respondents who lived alone and 3.3 per cent respondents who lived with spouse in the older group.

In conclusion, it was seen that saree/blouse/petticoat is the garment worn by the majority of the respondents, for any type of activity. The younger group respondents were more varied in the garments they wore as compared to the older group. Dress and trouser-top was not worn at all by the older group.

Variations Seen Corresponding to the Seasons

These have been represented in Tables 3A, 3B, 4A, 4B, 5A and 5B.

Summer

Colour: The colour preferred by most of the respondents was light/pastel colours, for all type of garments they wore. This was observed more in the younger group as compared to the older group. Dark and bright colours were also worn by a small percentage of respondents in the younger group and the percentage of respondents in the older group were more as compared to the younger group.

- A small number of respondents in the younger group said that no flashy/bright colours should be worn.
- A small number of respondents in both the groups had no specifications with respect to colour in the garments they wore.

Fabric: The fabric most preferred was cotton in both the groups.

- A small percentage of respondents in the younger group preferred to wear silk and synthetic fabric.
- A small percentage of respondents in the older group preferred to wear synthetic, Kota and hand-woven/khadi type of fabric in summers.

Print: The print preferred by both the groups was small/floral print, clear print and fine print irrespective of the garment. A small number of respondents did not prefer any print at all, which was more for blouse petticoat, saree and gown.

- Respondents who did not prefer any print were more in the older group as compared to the younger group.
- Small, floral or clear print was more preferred by younger group.

Winter

Colour: Colours preferred were dark, bright colours, followed by pastel/light colour.

- More number of respondents in the older group preferred light/pastel colours for saree, blouse and gown.
- More number of respondents in the younger group preferred dark, bright colours.
- Both the groups preferred light/pastel colours for gown.
- More respondents in younger group preferred not to wear flashy/bright coloured clothes.
- No specification was observed in younger group.

Fabric: Fabric preferred was cotton, silk, synthetic fabrics and woollens.

- More variation was found in younger group than older group.
- Younger group preferred cotton, silk synthetic fabrics for saree/blouse/petticoat, salwar-kameez, gown and trouser-top.

- Older group preferred cotton more than silk and synthetic for sarees/blouse/petticoat.
- More number of respondents in the older group had no specification than younger.

  Print: Again small, floral and fine print was preferred.
- In younger group small, floral and fine print was preferred for saree/blouse/petticoat and salwar-kameez and gown. For petticoat, a large number of respondents preferred plain. A small per cent of respondents preferred all type of prints/no specifications.
- In older group, small, floral print was preferred, followed by all types of print. More number of respondents in older group than younger group preferred no print/plain garments.

Monsoon

Colour: Colour preferred was light/pastel, followed by dark colour and bright colour.

- In the younger group light/pastel colours were preferred, followed by dark colour and bright colours. Only 12.2 per cent respondents preferred petticoats that matched with saree. A small percentage of respondents did not like black colour or flashy/bright colours.
- Few respondents had no specification about the colour they used.
- Less variation was observed in older group.
- Colours preferred were light/pastels, dark colours and bright colour.

Fabric: Fabric preferred was synthetic and cotton for saree, while cotton for blouse.

- In younger group, more respondents preferred synthetic fabric, followed by cotton and silk for saree, cotton for salwar-kameez and gown.
- In older group, respondents in equal numbers preferred cotton and synthetic fabric for saree. Cotton was preferred for blouse and gowns.
- *Print:* Print preferred was small print, followed by plain clothes.
- In the younger group, most of the respondents preferred clear print followed by small print.
- No print was also preferred by a large number of respondents in both groups.

Table 3 A *Variations in Colours*

Pattern	*Garments Living Arrange*	*Young-Old*																							
		Summer								*Winter*								*Monsoon*							
		A	*B*	*C*	*D*	*E*	*F*	*G*	*H*	*A*	*B*	*C*	*D*	*E*	*F*	*G*	*H*	*A*	*B*	*C*	*D*	*E*	*F*	*G*	*H*
Dark Colour	LA	6.7	3.3	3.3	—	—	—	—	—	6.7	—	—	—	—	—	3.3		6.7		3.3	—	—	—		—
	LS	10.0	10.0	13.3	—	—	—	10.0	3.3	40.0	31.0	30.0	16.7	6.7	—	10.0	—	20.0		23.3	6.7	3.3	—		3.3
	LF	10.0	13.3	10.0	3.3	—	—	10.0	—	23.3	23.3	20.0	6.7	—	—	6.7	—	20.0		20.0	3.3	—	—		—
	Total	8.9	8.9	8.9	1.1	—	—	6.7	1.1	23.3	18.0	16.7	7.8	2.2	—	6.7	—	15.6		15.6	3.3	1.1	—		1.1
Bright Colour	LA	6.7	3.3	3.3	—	—	—	—	10.0	3.3	3.3	3.3	—		—	—	—	3.3		3.3	—	—	—		3.3
	LS	10.0	10.0	3.3	—	—	—	3.3	16.7	3.3	10.3	—	3.3		—	3.3	6.7	3.3		—	6.7	—	3.3		3.3
	LF	10.0	10.0	3.3	3.3	—	—	6.7	6.7	20.0	20.0	16.7	3.3		—	3.3	3.3	16.7		13.3	3.3	—	—		—
	Total	8.9	7.8	10.0	1.1	—	—	3.3	11.1	8.9	11.2		2.2		—	2.2	—	7.8		5.6	3.3	—	1.1		2.2
Light/ Pastel	LA	26.7	26.7	5.6	3.3	3.3	—	6.7	--	26.7	30.0		3.3		—	6.7	3.3	26.7		30.0	—	—	—		
	LS	66.7	46.7	30.0	20.0	6.7	—	23.3	—	33.3	24.1		—		3.3	13.3	—	50.0		36.7	10.0	—	—		
	LF	46.7	40.0	40.0	10.0	—	—	20.0	3.3	33.3	30.0		6.7		—	16.7	—	36.7		20.0	10.0	—	—		
	Total	46.7	37.8	33.3	11.1	3.3	—	16.7	1.1	31.1	28.1		3.3		1.1	12.2	—	37.8		28.9	6.7	—	—		
Matching with saree	LA	—	3.3	34.4	—	—	—	—	—	—	3.3		—		—	—	—	—		—	3.3	—	—		
	LS	—	16.7	33.3	3.3	—	—	—	3.3	—	10.3		3.3		—	—	—	—		23.3	—	—	—		
	LF	3.3	6.7	13.3	—	—	—	—	6.7	3.3	3.3		—		—	—	—	3.3		13.3	—	—	—		
	Total	1.1	8.9	15.6	1.1	—	—	—	3.3	1.1	5.6		1.1		—	—	—	1.1		12.2	1.1	—	—		

Cont'd...

Cont'd...

		A	B	C	D	E	F	G	H	A	B	C	D	E	F	G	H	A	B	C	D	E	F	G	H
No Black Clothes	LA	3.3	3.3	3.3	—	—	—	—	—	3.3	3.3		—		—	—	—	3.3		3.3	—	—	—		
	LS	—	—	—	—	—	—	—	—	—	—		—		—	—	—	—		—	—	—	—		
	LF	—	—	—	—	—	—	—	—	—	—		—		—	—	—	—		—	—	—	—		
	Total	1.1	1.1	1.1	—	—	—	—	—	1.1	1.1		—		—	—	—	1.1		1.1	—	—	—		
No Flashy/ Bright	LA	—	—	—	—	—	—	—	—	—	—		—		—	—	—	—		—	—	—	—		
	LS	3.3	6.7	6.7	—	—	—	—	—	3.3	3.4		—		—	—	—	3.3		—	—	—	—		
	LF	6.7	6.7	6.7	—	—	—	—	—	6.7	6.7		—		—	—	—	6.7		6.7	—	—	—		
	Total	3.3	4.4	4.4	—	—	—	—	—	3.3	3.4		—		—	—	—	3.3		2.2	—	—	—		
No Specification	LA	3.3	3.3	3.3	3.3	3.3	3.3	3.3	—	3.3	3.3		3.3	3.3	3.3	3.3	3.3	3.3		3.3	3.3	3.3	3.3		3.3
	LS	3.3	3.3	3.3	—	—	—	—	3.3	13.3	13.8		—	—	—	—	—	16.7		13.3	—	—	—		—
	LF	10.0	6.7	6.7	—	—	—	—	6.7	13.3	13.3		—	—	—	3.3	—	16.7		13.3	—	—	—		—
	Total	5.6	4.4	4.4	1.2	1.1	1.1	1.1	3.3	10.0	10.1		1.1	1.1	1.1	2.2	1.1	12.2		10.0	1.1	1.1	1.1		1.1
NA	LA	56.7	60.0	60.0	93.3	93.3	96.7	90.0	90.0	60.0	60.0		93.3	96.7	96.7	90.0	93.3	60.0		60.0	93.3	96.7	96.7		193.3
	LS	10.0	10.0	10.0	76.7	93.3	100.0	63.3	73.3	10.0	10.3		76.7	93.3	96.7	76.7	96.7	10.0		10.0	80.0	96.7	96.7		193.3
	LF	33.3	36.7	40.0	90.0	100.0	100.0	73.3	83.3	33.3	36.7		90.0	100.0	100.0	76.7	100.0	33.3		40.0	90.0	100.0	100.0		200.0
	Total	33.3	35.6	36.7	86.7	95.6	100.0	75.6	82.2	34.4	36.0		86.7	96.7	97.8	81.1	96.7	34.4		36.7	87.8	97.8	97.8		195.6
NR	LA	—	—	—	—	—	—	—	3.3	—	—	—	—	—	—	—	—		—	—	—	—	—	—	—
	LS	—	—	—	—	—	—	—	6.6	—	—	—	—	—	—	—	—	—	—	—	—	—	—	—	—
	LF	—	—	—	—	—	—	—	6.6	—	—	—	—	—	—	—	—	—	—	—	—	—	—	—	—
	Total	—	—	—	—	—	—	—	5.6	—	—	—	—	—	—	—	—	—	—	—	—	—	—	—	—

A: Saree, B: Saree-Blouse, C: Saree-Petticoat, D: Salwar-Kameez, E: Dress, F: Trouser and Top, G: Gown, H: Any other, NA: Not Applicable, NR: No Response.

* Multiple Responses.

Table 3 B *Variations in Colours*

Pattern	Garments Living Arrange	Young -Old																							
		Summer								Winter								Monsoon							
		A	*B*	*C*	*D*	*E*	*F*	*G*	*H*	*A*	*B*	*C*	*D*	*E*	*F*	*G*	*H*	*A*	*B*	*C*	*D*	*E*	*F*	*G*	*H*
Dark Colour	LA	10.0	6.7	6.7	3.3			—	—	13.3	10.0		3.3			3.3	—	13.3		10.0	6.7				—
	LS	6.7	3.3	3.3	—			—	—	3.3	3.3		—			3.3	—	—		—	—				—
	LF	—	—	—	—			—	—	3.3	3.3		—			3.3	—	—		—	—				—
	Total	5.6	3.3	3.3	1.1			—	—	6.7	5.6		1.1			3.3	—	4.4		3.3	2.2				—
Bright Colour	LA	6.7	6.7	6.7	3.3			3.3	6.7	3.3	3.3		3.3			—	—	3.3		3.3	3.3				—
	LS	—	—	—	—			—	3.3	—	—		—			—	—	—		—	—				—
	LF	3.3	3.3	3.3	—			—	3.3	6.7	3.3		—			—	—	6.7		3.3	—				—
	Total	3.3	3.3	3.3	1.1			1.1	4.4	3.3	2.2		1.1			—	—	3.3		2.2	1.1				—
Light/ Patel	LA	26.7	23.3	23.3	6.7			6.7	—	23.3	20.0		6.7			6.7	—	26.7		23.3	3.3				—
	LS	13.3	10.0	13.3	3.3			6.7	—	16.7	10.0		3.3			3.3	—	16.7		13.3	3.3				—
	LF	43.3	40.0	43.3	—			10.0	—	33.3	36.7		—			6.7	—	40.0		40.0	—				—
	Total	27.8	24.4	26.7	3.3			7.8	—	24.4-	22.2		3.3			5.6	—	27.8		25.6	2.2				—
Matching with saree	LA	—	—	—	—			—	—	—			—			—	—	—		—	—				—
	LS	—	—	—	—			—	—	—			—			—	—	—		—	—				—
	LF	—	3.3	—	—			—	—	—			—			—	—	—		—	—				—
	Total	—	1.1	—	—			—	—	—			—			—	—	—		—	—				—

Cont'd...

Cont'd...

		A	*B*	*C*	*D*	*E*	*F*	*G*	*H*	*A*	*B*	*C*	*D*	*E*	*F*	*G*	*H*	*A*	*B*	*C*	*D*	*E*	*F*	*G*	*H*
No Black Clothes	LA	—	—	—	—			—	—	—			—			—	—	—		—	—				—
	LS	—	—	—	—			—	—	—			—			—	—	—		—	—				—
	LF	—	—	—	—			—	—	3.3			—			—	—	—		—	—				—
	Total	—	—	—	—			—	—	1.1			—			—	—	—		—	—				—
No Flashy/ Bright	LA	—	—	—	—			—	—	3.3	3.3		—			—	—	—		—	—				—
	LS	—	—	—	—			—	—	—	—		—			—	—	—		—	—				—
	LF	—	—	—	—			—	—	—	—		—			—	—	—		—	—				—
	Total	—	—	—	—			—	—	1.1	1.1		—			—	—	—		—	—				—
No Specification	LA	—	—	—	—			—	—	—	—		—			—	—	—		—	—				—
	LS	6.7	6.7	3.3	—			3.3		6.7	6.7		—			3.3	—	10.0		10.0	—				—
	LF	—	—	—	—			—	3.3	—	—		—			—	—	—		—	—				—
	Total	2.2	2.2	1.1	—			1.1	1.1	2.2	2.2		—			1.1	—	3.3		3.3	—				—
NA	LA	73.3	76.7	76.7	93.3			93.3	93.3	73.3	76.7		93.3			93.3	100.0	73.3		76.7	93.3				200.0
	LS	73.3	80.0	80.0	96.7			90.0	90.0	73.3	80.0		96.7			90.0	100.0	73.3		76.7	96.7				200.0
	LF	53.3	53.3	53.3	100.0			90.0	90.0	53.3	56.7		100.0			90.0	100.0	53.3		56.7	100.0				200.0
	Total	66.7	70.0	70.0	96.7			91.1	91.1	66.7	71.1		96.7			91.1	100.0	66.7		70.0	96.7				200.0
NR	LA	—	—	—	—	—	—	—	6.7	—	—	—	—	—	—	—	—		—	—	—	—	—	—	—
	LS	—	—	—	—	—	—	—	6.7	—	—	—	—	—	—	—	—	—	—	—	—	—	—	—	—
	LF	—	—	—	—	—	—	—	3.3	—	—	—	—	—	—	—	—	—	—	—	—	—	—	—	—
	Total	—	—	—	—	—	—	—	5.6	—	—	—	—	—	—	—	—	—	—	—	—	—	—	—	—

A: Saree, B: Saree-Blouse, C: Saree-Petticoat, D: Salwar-Kameez, E: Dress, F: Trouser and Top, G: Gown, H: Any other, NA: Not Applicable, NR: No Response

* Multiple Responses

Table 4 A *Variations in Fabric*

Pattern	*Garments Living Arrange*	*Young-Old*																							
		Summer								*Winter*								*Monsoon*							
		A	*B*	*C*	*D*	*E*	*F*	*G*	*H*	*A*	*B*	*C*	*D*	*E*	*F*	*G*	*H*	*A*	*B*	*C*	*D*	*E*	*F*	*G*	*H*
Cotton	LA	40.0	40.0	40.0	6.7	6.7	3.3	10.0	—	16.7	23.3	33.3	3.3	—	—	3.3				30.0	3.3	—	—	—	
	LS	86.7	70.0	80.0	23.3	6.7	—	33.3	—	16.7	26.7	56.7	6.7	—	3.3	10.0				73.3	10.0	3.3	3.3	6.7	
	LF	60.0	56.7	60.0	10.0	—	1.1	26.7	—	10.0	13.3	40.0	3.3	—	—	10.0				43.3	6.7	—	—	6.7	
	Total	62.2	55.6	60.0	13.3	4.4	—	23.3	—	14.4	21.1	43.3	4.4	—	1.1	7.8				48.9	6.7	1.1	1.1	4.4	
Silk	LA	—	—	—	—	—	—	—	—	16.7	6.7	6.7	3.3	3.3	3.3	3.3				6.7	3.3	3.3	3.3	—	
	LS	—	6.7	3.3	3.3	—	—	3.3	—	33.3	20.0	13.3	3.3	—	—	3.3				3.3	3.3	—	—	3.3	
	LF	—	—	—	—	—	—	—	—	20.0	16.7	6.7	—	—	—	3.3				10.0	—	—	—	3.3	
	Total	—	2.2	1.1	1.1	—	—	1.1	—	23.3	14.4	8.9	2.2	1.1	1.1	3.3				6.7	2.2	1.1	1.1	2.2	
Synthetic Fibre	LA	—	—	—	—	—	—	—	3.3	26.7	23.3	13.3	3.3	3.3	3.3	6.7				13.3	3.3	3.3	3.3	3.3	
	LS	3.3	—	3.3	3.3	—	—	—	3.3	40.0	33.3	10.0	6.7	3.3	—	10.0				16.7	3.3	—	—	16.7	
	LF	3.3	3.3	—	—	—	—	—	—	33.3	33.3	10.0	3.3	—	—	6.7				10.0	3.3	—	—	16.7	
	Total	2.2	1.1	1.1	1.1	—	—	—	2.2	33.3	30.0	11.1	4.4	2.2	1.1	7.8				13.3	3.3	1.1	1.1	12.2	
Terrycoat	LA	—	—	—	—	—	—	—	—	—	—	—	—	—	—	—				—	—	—	—	3.3-	
	LS	—	6.7	—	—	—	—	3.3	—	16.7	16.7	6.7	10.0	6.7	—	—				—	3.3	—	—	—	
	LF	—	—	—	—	—	—	3.3	—	—	—	3.3	—	—	—	—				6.7	—	—	—	1.1	
	Total	—	2.2	—	—	—	—	—	—	5.6	5.6	3.3	3.3	2.2	—	—				2.2	1.1	—	—	—	

Cont'd...

Cont'd...

		A	B	C	D	E	F	G	H	A	B	C	D	E	F	G	H	A	B	C	D	E	F	G	H
Kota	LA	—	—	—	—	—	—	2.2	—	—	—	—	—	—	—	—				—	—	—	—	—	
	LS	—	—	—	—	—	—	—	—	—	—	—	—	—	—	—				—	—	—	—	—	
	LF	—	—	—	—	—	—	—	—	—	—	—	—	—	—	—				—	—	—	—	—	
	Total	—	—	—	—	—	—	—	—	—	—	—	—	—	—	—				—	—	—	—	—	
Hand woven/ khadi	LA	—	—	—	—	—	—	—	—	—	—	—	—	—	—	—				—	—	—	—	—	
	LS	—	—	—	—	—	—	—	—	—	3.3	—	—	—	—	—				—	—	—	—	—	
	LF	—	—	—	—	—	—	—	—	—	—	3.3	—	—	—	—				—	—	—	—	—	
	Total	—	—	—	—	—	—	—	—	—	1.1	1.1	—	—	—	—				—	—	—	—	—	
Chan-deri	LA	—	—	—	—	—	—	—	3.3	—	—	—	—	—	—	—				—	—	—	—	3.3	
	LS	—	—	—	—	—	—	—	—	—	—	—	3.3	—	—	—				—	—	—	—	—	
	LF	—	—	—	—	—	—	—	—	—	—	—	—	—	—	—				—	—	—	—	—	
	Total	—	—	—	—	—	—	—	1.1	—	—	—	1.1	—	—	—				—	—	—	—	1.1	
Woollen	LA	—	—	—	—	—	—	—	—	3.3	6.7	—	—	—	—	—				—	—	—	—	—	
	LS	—	3.3	3.3	—	—	—	—	—	3.3	6.7	6.7	—	—	—	—				3.3		—	—	—	
	LF	—	—	—	—	—	—	—	—	3.3	3.3	—	3.3	—	—	—				3.3	3.3	—	—	—	
	Total	—	1.1	1.1	—	—	—	—	—	3.3	5.6	2.2	1.1	—	—	—				2.2	1.1	—	—	—	
Chiffon	LA	—	—	—	—	—	—	—	—	—	—	—	—	—	—	—				—	—	—	—	—	
	LS	—	—	—	—	—	—	—	—	—	—	—	—	—	—	—				—	—	—	—	—	
	LF	—	—	—	—	—	—	—	—	3.3	—	—	—	—	—	—				—	—	—	—	—	
	Total	—	—	—	—	—	—	—	—	1.1	—	—	—	—	—	—				—	—	—	—	—	

Cont'd...

Cont'd...

		A	B	C	D	E	F	G	H	A	B	C	D	E	F	G	H	A	B	C	D	E	F	G	H
Crepe	LA	—		—	—	—	—	—	—	—	—	—	—	—	—	—				—	—	—	—	—	
	LS	3.3	3.3	—	—	—	—	—	—	—	—	—	—	—	—	—				—	—	—	—	—	
	LF	—	—	—	—	—	—	—	—	—	—	—	—	—	—	—				—	—	—	—	—	
	Total	1.1	1.1	—	—	—	—	—	—	—	—	—	—	—	—	—				—	—	—	—	—	
Thick Fabric	LA	—	—	—	—	—	—	—	—	—	—	—	—	—	—	—				—	—	—	—	—	
	LS	—	—	—	—	—	—	—	—	3.3	—	—	—	—	—	—				—	—	—	—	—	
	LF	—	—	—	—	—	—	—	—	6.7	6.7	—	—	—	—	—				—	—	—	—	—	
	Total	—	—	—	—	—	—	—	—	3.3	2.2	—	—	—	—	—				—	—	—	—	—	
Light in weight	LA	—	—	—	—	—	—	—	—	—	—	—	—	—	—	—				—	—	—	—	—	
	LS	—	—	—	—	—	—	—	—	—	—	—	—	—	—	—				—	—	—	—	—	
	LF	3.3	3.3	—	—	—	—	—	—	—	—	—	—	—	—	—				—	—	—	—	—	
	Total	1.1	1.1	—	—	—	—	—	—	—	—	—	—	—	—	—				—	—	—	—	—	
NA	LA	60.0	60.0	60.0	93.3	93.3	96.7	90.0	93.3	60.0	60.0	60.0	93.3	96.7	96.7	90.0				60.0	93.3	96.7	96.7	90.0	
	LS	10.0	10.0	10.0	76.7	93.3	100.0	63.3	96.7	0.0	10.0	10.0	76.7	93.3	96.7	76.7				10.0	80.0	96.7	96.7	76.7	
	LF	33.3	36.7	40.0	90.0	100.0	100.0	73.3	100.0	3.3	36.7	40.0	90.0	100.0	100.0	76.7				40.0	90.0	100.0	100.0	80.0	
	Total	34.4	35.6	36.7	86.7	95.6	96.9	75.6	96.7	4.4	35.6	36.7	86.7	96.7	97.8	81.1				36.7	87.8	97.8	97.8	82.2	

A: Saree, B: Saree-Blouse, C: Saree-Petticoat, D: Salwar-Kameez, E: Dress, F: Trouser and Top, G: Gown, H: Any other, NA: Not Applicable, NR: No Response

* Multiple Responses

NA: No specification + respondents not wearing the particular garments.

Table 4 B *Variations in Fabric*

Pattern	Garments Living Arrange	Old-Old																							
		Summer								Winter								Monsoon							
		A	B	C	D	E	F	G	H	A	B	C	D	E	F	G	H	A	B	C	D	E	F	G	H
Cotton	LA	26.7	23.3	23.3	6.7			6.7		13.3		13.3	—	—	—	3.3	—			16.7	—	—	—	3.3	—
	LS	23.3	20.0	23.3	3.3			10.0		10.0		20.0	3.3	—	—	10.0	—			23.3	3.3	—	—	3.3	3.3
	LF	43.3	43.3	46.7	—			10.0		16.7		33.3	—	—	—	6.7	—			33.3	—	—	—	3.3	—
	Total	31.1	28.9	31.1	3.3			8.9		13.3		22.2	1.1	—	—	6.7	—			24.4	1.1	—	—	3.3	1.1
Silk	LA	—	—	—	—			—		6.7		6.7	3.3	—	—	3.3	—			6.7	3.3	—	—	—	—
	LS	—	—	—	—			—		10.0		3.3	—	—	—	—	—			—	—	—	—	—	—
	LF	—	—	—	—			—		16.7		3.3	—	—	—	—	—			6.7	—	—	—	—	—
	Total	—	—	—	—			—		11.1		4.4	1.1	—	—	1.1	—			4.4	1.1	—	—	—	—
Synthetic Fibre	LA	—	—	—	—			—		6.7		3.3	6.7	—	—	—	—			3.3	6.7	—	—	6.7	—
	LS	—	—	—	—			—		13.3		3.3	—	—	—	—	—			—	—	—	—	3.3	—
	LF	3.3	—	—	—			—		20.0		6.7	—	—	—	3.3	—			6.7	—	—	—	6.7	—
	Total	1.1	—	—	—			—		13.3		4.4	2.2	—	—	1.1	—			3.3	2.2	—	—	5.6	—
Terrycoat	LA	—	—	—	—			—		6.7		3.3	—	—	—	3.3	—			—	—	—	—	—	—
	LS	—	—	—	—			—		—		—	—	—	—	—	—			—	—	—	—	—	—
	LF	—	—	—	—			—		3.3		—	—	—	—	—	—			—	—	—	—	—	—
	Total	—	—	—	—			—		3.3		1.1	—	—	—	1.1	—			—	—	—	—	—	—

Cont'd...

Cont'd...

		A	*B*	*C*	*D*	*E*	*F*	*G*	*H*	*A*	*B*	*C*	*D*	*E*	*F*	*G*	*H*	*A*	*B*	*C*	*D*	*E*	*F*	*G*	*H*
Kota	LA	—	—	—	—			—					—	—	—	—	—			—	—	—	—	—	—
	LS	3.3	—	—	—			—					—	—	—	—	—			—	—	—	—	—	—
	LF	—	—	—	—			—					—	—	—	—	—			—	—	—	—	—	—
	Total	1.1	—	—	—			—					—	—	—	—	—			3.3	—	—	—	—	—
Hand woven/ khadi	LA	3.3	3.3	3.3	—			—					—	—	—	—	—			—	—	—	—	—	—
	LS	3.3		—	—			—		—			—	—	—	—	—			—	—	—	—	—	—
	LF	—		—	—			—		3.3			—	—	—	—	—			1.1	—	—	—	—	—
	Total	2.2	1.1	1.1	—			—		—			—	—	—	—	—			—	—	—	—	—	—
Chanderi	LA	—	—	—	—			—		1.1			—	—	—	—	—			—	—	—	—	—	—
	LS	—	—	—	—			—		—		3.3	—	—	—	—	—			—	—	—	—	—	—
	LF	—	—	—	—			—		—		—	—	—	—	—	—			—	—	—	—	6.7	—
	Total	—	—	—	—			—		—		1.1	—	—	—	—	—			—	—	—	—	—	—
Woollen	LA	—	—	—	—			—		—		—	—	—	—	—	—			—	—	—	—	2.2	—
	LS	—	—	—	—			—		6.7		—	—	—	—	—	—			—	—	—	—	—	—
	LF	—	—	—	—			—		—		—	—	—	—	—	—			—	—	—	—	—	—
	Total	—	—	—	—			—		—		—	—	—	—	—	—			3.3	—	—	—	—	—
Chiffon	LA	—	—	—	—			—		2.2		—	—	—	—	—	—			1.1	—	—	—	—	—
	LS	—	—	—	—			—		—		—	—	—	—	—	—			—	—	—	—	—	—
	LF	—	—	—	—			—		—		—	—	—	—	—	—			—	—	—	—	—	—
	Total	—	—	—	—			—		—		—	—	—	—	—	—			—	—	—	—	—	—

Cont'd...

Cont'd...

		A	B	C	D	E	F	G	H	A	B	C	D	E	F	G	H	A	B	C	D	E	F	G	H
Crepe	LA	—	—	—	—			—	—	—		—	—	—	—	—	—			—	—	—	—	—	—
	LS	—	—	—	—			—	—	—		—	—	—	—	—	—			—	—	—	—	—	—
	LF	—	—	—	—			—	—	—		—	—	—	—	—	—			—	—	—	—	—	—
	Total	—	—	—	—			—	—	—		—	—	—	—	—	—			—	—	—	—	—	—
Thick Fabric	LA	—	—	—	—			—	—	—		—	—	—	—	—	—			—	—	—	—	—	—
	LS	—	—	—	—			—	—	—		—	—	—	—	—	—			—	—	—	—	—	—
	LF	—	—	—	—			—	—	3.3		3.3	—	—	—	—	—			—	—	—	—	—	—
	Total	—	—	—	—			—	—	1.1		1.1	—	—	—	—	—			—	—	—	—	—	—
Light in weight	LA	—	—	—	—			—	—	—		—	—	—	—	—	—			—	—	—	—	—	—
	LS	—	—	—	—			—	—	—		—	—	—	—	—	—			—	—	—	—	—	—
	LF	—	—	—	—			—	—	—		—	—	—	—	—	—			—	—	—	—	—	—
	Total	—	—	—	—			—	—	—		—	—	—	—	—	—			—	—	—	—	—	—
NA	LA	73.3	76.7	76.7	93.3			93.3	100.0	73.3		76.7	93.3	100.0	100.0	93.3	100.0			76.7	93.3	100.0	100.0	93.3	100.0
	LS	73.3	80.0	76.7	96.7			90.0	100.0	73.3		76.7	96.7	100.0	100.0	90.0	100.0			76.7	96.7	100.0	100.0	90.0	96.7
	LF	53.3	53.3	53.3	100.0			90.0	100.0	53.3		56.7	100.0	100.0	100.0	90.0	100.0			56.7	100.0	100.0	100.0	90.0	100.0
	Total	66.7	70.0	68.9	96.7			91.1	100.0	66.7		70.0	96.7	100.0	100.0	91.1	100.0			70.0	96.7	100.0	100.0	91.1	98.9

A: Saree, B: Saree-Blouse, C: Saree-Petticoat, D: Salwar-Kameez, E: Dress, F: Trouser and Top, G: Gown, H: Any other, NA: Not Applicable, NR: No Response

* Multiple Responses

NA: No specification + respondents not wearing the particular garments.

Table 5A *Variation in Print*

Pattern	*Garments Living Arrange*	*Young -Old*																							
		Summer								*Winter*								*Monsoon*							
		A	*B*	*C*	*D*	*E*	*F*	*G*	*H*	*A*	*B*	*C*	*D*	*E*	*F*	*G*	*H*	*A*	*B*	*C*	*D*	*E*	*F*	*G*	*H*
Clear print	LA	6.7	6.7	6.7	—	—	—	—	6.7	6.7	6.7	6.7	—	—	—	—				6.7	—	—	—	3.3	
	LS	6.7	—	—	3.3	—	—	3.3	3.3	6.7	10.0	6.7	6.7	3.3	3.3	—				10.0	3.3		6.7	13.3	
	LF	—	—	—	—	—	—	—	—	—	—	—	—	—	—	—				—	—		—	10.0	
	Total	4.4	2.2	2.2	1.1	—	—	1.1	3.3	4.4	5.6	4.4	2.2	1.1	1.1	—				5.6	1.1		2.2	8.9	
Small/ Floral-print	LA	26.7	20.0	13.3	3.3	6.7	3.3	6.7	—	26.7	26.7	13.3	3.3	3.3	3.3	6.7	3.3			16.7	6.7	3.3	3.3	3.3	
	LS	60.0	43.3	6.7	10.0	3.3	—	20.0	—	53.3	46.7	10.0	10.0	3.3	—	20.0	—			6.7	10.0	3.3		—	
	LF	33.3	30.0	10.0	6.7	—	—	16.7	—	36.7	33.3	13.3	3.3	—	—	13.3	—			16.7	3.3	—		6.7	
	Total	40.0	31.1	10.0	6.7	3.3	1.1	14.4	—	38.9	35.6	12.2	5.6	2.2	1.1	13.3	1.1			13.3	6.7	2.2	1.1	3.3	
Small/ Fine print	LA	3.3	3.3	3.3	—	—	—	—	—	3.3	3.3	6.7	—	—	—	3.3	3.3			—	—	—	—	6.7	
	LS	6.7	—	3.3	—	—	—	—	—	10.0	3.3	13.3	—	—	—	—	3.3			3.3	—	—	--	6.7	
	LF	10.0	6.7	—	—	—	—	—	—	10.0	3.3	3.3	—	—	—	—	—			—	—	—	—	6.7	
	Total	6.7	3.3	2.2					—	7.8	3.3	7.8				1.1	2.2			1.1				6.7	
Medium print.	LA	—	—	—	—	—	—	—	—	—	—	—	—	—	—	—	—			—	—	—	—	—	
	LS	3.3	10.0	—	—	—	—	—	—	6.7	6.7	—	—	—	—	—	—			—	—	—	—	6.7	
	LF	—	—	—	—	—	—	—	—	—	—	—	—	—	—	—	—			—	—	—	—	—	
	Total	1.1	3.3	—	—	—	—	—	—	2.2	2.2													2.2	

Cont'd...

Cont'd...

		A	B	C	D	E	F	G	H	A	B	C	D	E	F	G	H	A	B	C	D	E	F	G	H
Border in print	LA	—		—	—	—	—	—	—	—	—	—	—	—	—	—	—			—	—	—	—	—	
	LS	—		—	—	—	—	—	—	—	—	—	—	—	—	—	—			—	—	—	—	—	
	LF	3.3		—	—	—	—	—	—	—		—	—	—	—	—	—			—	—	—	—	—	
	Total	1.1		—	—	—	—	—	—	—	—	—	—	—	—	—	—			—	—	—	—		
Block print	LA	—		—	—	—	—	—	—	—	—	—	—	—	—	—	—			—	—	—	—	—	
	LS	—		—	—	—	—	—	—	—	—	—	—	—	—	—	—			—	—	—	—	—	
	LF	3.3	3.3	3.3	—	—	—	—	—	3.3	3.3	3.3	—	—	—	—	—			3.3	—	—	—	—	
	Total	1.1	1.1	1.1	—	—	—	—	—	1.1	1.1	1.1	—	—	—	—	—			1.1	—	—	—	—	
All types of print	LA	—	—	—	—	—	—	—	—	—	—	—	—	—	—	—	—			—	—	—	—	—	
	LS	6.7	3.3	3.3	—	—	—	3.3	—	10.0	6.7	6.7	3.3	—	—	3.3	—			6.7				—	
	LF	16.7	16.7	10.0	3.3	—	—	6.7	—	16.7	16.7	6.7	3.3	—	—	6.7	—			10.0	3.3	—	—	—	
	Total	7.8	6.7	4.4	1.1	—	—	3.3	—	8.9	7.8	4.4	2.2	—	—	3.3	—			5.6	1.1	—	—	—	
No Print/ plain	LA	23.3	30.0	36.7	6.7	3.3	3.3	6.7	—	20.0	20.0	30.0	6.7	3.3	3.3	3.3				26.7	3.3	3.3	3.3	—	
	LS	13.3	36.7	80.0	10.0	—	—	10.0	—	6.7	20.0	53.3	3.3	—	—	3.3	—			66.7	3.3	—	3.3		
	LF	6.7	13.3	43.3	—	—	—	6.7	—	6.7	13.3	40.0	3.3	—	—	6.7	—			36.7	3.3	—	—	3.3	
	Total	14.4	26.7	53.3	5.6	1.1	1.1	7.8	—	11.1	17.8	41.1	4.4	1.1	1.1	4.4	—			43.3	3.3	1.1	2.2	1.1	
NA	LA	60.0	60.0	60.0	93.3	93.3	96.7	90.0	93.3	60.0	60.0	60.0	93.3	96.7	96.7	90.0	96.7			60.0	93.3	96.7	96.7	90.0	
	LS	10.0	10.0	10.0	76.7	96.7	100.0	66.7	96.7	10.0	10.0	13.3	76.7	93.3	96.7	76.7	96.7			10.0	83.3	96.7	90.0	76.7	
	LF	33.3	36.7	40.0	90.0	100.0	100.0	73.3	100.0	33.3	36.7	40.0	90.0	100.0	100.0	76.7	100.0			40.0	90.0	100.0	100.0	80.0	
	Total	34.4	35.6	36.7	86.7	96.7	98.9	76.7	96.7	34.4	35.6	37.8	86.7	96.7	97.8	81.1	97.8			36.7	88.9	97.8	95.6	82.2	

A: Saree, B: Saree-Blouse, C: Saree-Petticoat, D: Salwar-Kameez, E: Dress, F: Trouser and Top, G: Gown, H: Any other, NA: Not Applicable, NR: No Response.

* Multiple Responses.

Table 5B *Variation in Print*

Pattern	Garments Living Arrange	Old-Old																							
		Summer								Winter								Monsoon							
		A	B	C	D	E	F	G	H	A	B	C	D	E	F	G	H	A	B	C	D	E	F	G	H
Clear print	LA	—				—	—	—		3.3	3.3	3.3	—	—	—		—			—	—	—	—	3.3	
	LS	3.3	6.7	—	3.3	—	—	—		3.3	6.7	6.7	—	—	—		—			6.7	—	—	—	10.0	
	LF	6.7	10.0	6.7	—	—	—	—		6.7	6.7	10.0	—	—	—		—			6.7	—	—	—	6.7	
	Total	3.3	5.6	2.2	1.1	—	—	—		4.4	5.6	6.7	—	—	—		—			4.4	—	—	—	6.7	
Small/ Floral print	LA	23.3	16.7	16.7	—	—	—	6.7		20.0	13.3	13.3	—	—	—	6.7	—			13.3	—	—	—	6.7	
	LS	13.3	6.7	3.3	—	—	—	3.3		13.3	10.0	3.3	—	—	—	3.3	—			6.7	3.3	—	—	—	
	LF	23.3	23.3	13.3	—	—	—	6.7		23.3	23.3	13.3	—	—	—	3.3	—			10.0	—	—	—	—	
	Total	20.0	15.6	11.1	—	—	—	5.6		18.9	15.6	10.0	—	—	—	4.4	—			10.0	1.1	—	—	2.2	
Small/ Fine print	LA	—	—	—	—	—	—	—		3.3	3.3	3.3	—	—	—		—			—	—	—	—	—	
	LS	—	—	—	—	—	—	—		—	—	—	—	—	—		—			—	—	—	—	—	
	LF	3.3	3.3	—	—	—	—	—		6.7	6.7	—	—	—	—		—			—	—	—	—	3.3	
	Total	1.1	1.1	—	—	—	—	—		3.3	3.3	1.1	—	—	—		—			—	—	—	—	1.1	
Medium print	LA	—	—	—	—	—	—	—		—	—						—			—	—	—	—	—	
	LS	—	—	3.3	—	—	—	—		—	—	—	—	—	—	—	—			—	—	—	—	—	
	LF	—	—	—	—	—	—	—		3.3	—	—	—	—	—	—	—			—	—	—	—	—	
	Total	—	—	1.1	—	—	—	—		1.1	—	—	—	—	—	—	—			—	—	—	—	—	
Border in print	LA	—	—	—	—	—	—	—		—	—	—	—	—	—	—	—			—	—	—	—	—	
	LS	—	—	—	—	—	—	—		—	—	—	—	—	—	—	—			—	—	—	—	—	
	LF	—	—	—	—	—	—	—		—	—	—	—	—	—	—	—			—	—	—	—	—	
	Total	—	—	—	—	—	—	—		—	—	—	—	—	—	—	—			—	—	—	—	—	

Cont'd...

Cont'd...

		A	B	C	D	E	F	G	H	A	B	C	D	E	F	G	H	A	B	C	D	E	F	G	H
Block print	LA	—	—	—	—	—	—	—		—	—	—	—	—	—	—	—			—	—	—	—	—	
	LS	—	—	—	—	—	—	—		—	—	—	—	—	—	—	—			—	—	—	—	—	
	LF	—	—	—	—	—	—	—		—	—	—	—	—	—	—	—			—	—	—	—	—	
	Total	—	-	—	—	—	—	—		—	—	—	—	—	—	—	—			—	—	—	—	—	
All types of print	LA	3.3	3.3	—	3.3	—	—	—		3.3	3.3		3.3	—	—	—	—			—	3.3	—	—	—	
	LS	—	—	—	—	—	—	—		—	—		—	—	—	—	—			—	—	—	—	—	
	LF	—	—	—	—	—	—	—		—	—		—	—	—	3.3	—			—	—	—	—	—	
	Total	1.1	1.1	—	1.1	—	—	—		1.1	1.1		1.1	—	—	1.1	—			—	1.1	—	—	—	
No Print/ plain	LA	13.3	16.7	20.0	3.3	—	—	6.7		10.0	13.3	16.7	3.3	—	—	6.7	—			20.0	3.3	—	—	—	
	LS	20.0	16.7	20.0	—	—	—	6.7		20.0	13.3	20.0	3.3	—	—	6.7	—			16.7	—	—	—	—	
	LF	20.0	16.7	30.0	—	—	—	—		13.3	13.3	23.3	—	—	—	—	—			30.0	—	—	—	—	
	Total	17.8	16.7	23.3	1.1	—	—	4.4		14.4	13.3	20.0	2.2	—	—	4.4	—			22.2	1.1	—	—	—	
NA	LA	73.3	76.7	76.7	93.3	100.0	100.0	93.3		73.3	76.7	76.7	93.3	100.0	100.0	93.3	—			76.7	—	100.0	100.0	93.3	
	LS	73.3	80.0	76.7	96.7	100.0	100.0	90.0		73.3	80.0	76.7	96.7	100.0	100.0	90.0	—			76.7	—	100.0	100.0	90.0	
	LF	53.3	56.7	56.7	100.0	100.0	100.0	90.0		53.3	56.7	56.7	100.0	100.0	100.0	90.0	3.3			56.7	—	100.0	100.0	90.0	
	Total	66.7	71.1	70.0	96.7	100.0	100.0	91.1		66.7	70.0	70.0	96.7	100.0	100.0	91.1	1.1			70.0	—	100.0	100.0	91.1	
NR	LA	—	—	—	—	—	—	—		—	—	—	3.3	—	—	—	—			—	93.3	—	—	—	
	LS	—	—	—	—	—	—	—		—	—	—	—	—	—	—	—			—	96.7	—	—	—	
	LF	3.3	3.3	3.3	—	—	—	3.3		—	—	3.3	—	—	—	3.3	—			3.3	100.0	—	—	—	
	Total	1.1	1.1	1.1	—	—	—	1.1		—	—	1.1	1.1	—	—	1.1	—			1.1	96.7	—	—	—	

A: Saree, B: Saree-Blouse, C: Saree-Petticoat, D: Salwar-Kameez, E: Dress, F: Trouser and Top, G: Gown, H: Any other, NA: Not Applicable, NR: No Response

* Multiple Responses

Garments do not Vary with Season

As shown in Table 6 the major reasons given for garments not varying with seasons were that respondents liked to wear all types of fabrics in all seasons, wear what was available to them and silk fabric is meant only to be worn for occasions.

- More number of respondents in the older group than younger group said that they liked to wear all types of fabrics, colours and print in all seasons, i.e., they have no specifications for their wardrobe. The maximum number of respondents fall in the living alone category in both the groups (44.8% YO and 43.3% OO). In the younger group the living alone respondents are followed by living with family (20%) and living with spouse (6.7%). In the older group living alone respondents are followed by respondents living with spouse (33.3%) and living with family (26.7%).

Table 6 *Garments do not Vary with Season*

Respondents' Reasons	*Young-Old*				*Old-Old*				*Total N*
	LA	*LS*	*LF*	*Total*	*LA*	*LS*	*LF*	*Total*	
Wear all types of colour print and fabric	44.8	6.7	20.0	23.6	43.3	33.3	26.7	34.4	29.5
Wear what is available	24.1	—	—	7.9	10.0	43.3	16.7	23.3	15.6
Silk only for occasions	3.4	3.3	10.0	5.6	6.7	10.0	3.3	6.7	6.15
Like to wear synthetics	3.4	3.3	10.0	5.6	6.7	—	6.7	4.4	
Wear only cotton and specific colour	—	—	—	—	13.3	3.3	10.0	8.9	4.45
Wear what is suitable to my skin type	3.4	—	3.3	2.2	—	6.7	—	2.2	2.2
Medical reasons	3.4	—	—	1.1	—	3.3	3.3	2.2	1.65
NA	41.4	86.7	66.7	65.2	30.0	30.0	46.7	35.6	

Table shows multiple responses.

- About 15.6 per cent respondents wore what was available to them. This was seen more in older respondents (23.3%), than younger respondents (7.9%). In the younger group respondents were present only in living alone category (24.1%). In the older group the maximum response was from respondents living with spouse followed by respondents who lived with family and lastly respondents living alone.
- Silk was worn only for occasion like festivals, by 6.7 per cent respondents in older group and 5.6 per cent respondents in younger group. In the younger group, maximum response was obtained from respondents who lived alone (10%), followed by respondents who lived with spouse with very minimal difference between the two. In the older group, the maximum number of responses was obtained from respondents living with spouse (10%), followed by respondents living alone and lastly respondents living with family.
- Only 5 per cent of respondents in both the groups, with a marginal difference between the two like to wear synthetic clothes for all seasons. This was seen in more number in respondents who lived with family (10%) followed by equal number of respondent in other two categories, i.e., respondents living alone and respondents living with spouse in the younger group. In the older group, it was seen in equal per cent of respondents in living alone and living with family categories.
- About 8.9 per cent in the older group wore only cotton fabric and a special colour. This was seen more in respondents living alone (13.3%) and respondents who lived with family (10%), as compared to respondents who lived with spouse (3.3%) only. There was no response in the younger group.
- Just only 2,2 per cent respondents in both the groups wore what was suitable to their respective skin types. In the younger group it was seen in equal number of respondents who lived alone and lived with family. In the older group 6.7 per cent respondents who lived with spouse were there only.
- Merely 2.2. per cent respondents in older group gave the reason for garments not varying with season, as medical reason. There were an equal number of respondents in living with spouse and living with family category. 3.4 per cent respondents who lived alone in younger group also gave medical reason for garments not varying with season.

Table 7 *Clothing Preference*

Pattern	Garments Living Arrange	Young-Old								Old-Old							
		A	B	C	D	E	F	G	H	A	B	C	D	E	F	G	H
Hand-Made	LA	6.7	—	—	—	—	—	—	—	—	3.3	6.7	—	—	—	—	—
	LS	16.7	16.7	13.3	—	—	—	—	—	3.3	6.7	6.7	3.3	10.0	6.7	3.3	—
	LF	10.0	—	3.3	—	—	—	—	—	3.3	3.3	—	—	—	—	—	—
	Total	11.1	5.6	5.8	—	—	—	—	—	2.2	4.4	4.4	1.1	3.3	2.2	1.1	—
Tailor-Made	LA	—	60.0	16.7	6.7	—	—	3.3	6.7	—	63.3	26.7	3.3	—	—	6.7	6.7
	LS	—	73.3	26.7	13.3	—	—	13.3	—	—	56.7	16.7	6.7	3.3	—	6.7	3.3
	LF	—	70.0	23.3	3.3	3.3	—	3.3	—	—	53.3	23.3	—	—	—	3.3	—
	Total	—	67.8	22.2	7.8	1.1	—	6.7	2.2	—	57.8	22.2	3.3	1.1	—	5.6	3.3
Ready-Made	LA	80.0	3.3	60.0	—	—	—	16.7	6.7	90.0	—	50.0	6.7	—	—	20.0	3.3
	LS	83.3	—	43.3	10.0	3.3	3.3	33.3	—	90.0	6.7	63.3	3.3	—	—	20.0	—
	LF	86.7	—	56.7	6.7	3.3	—	23.3	—	90.0	—	63.3	—	—	—	6.7	—
	Total	83.3	1.1	53.3	5.6	2.2	1.1	24.4	2.2	90.0	2.2	58.9	3.3	—	—	15.6	1.1
Ready-Made and Tailor-Made	LA	—	26.7	6.7	10.0	3.3	3.3	3.3	6.7	—	23.3	6.7	—	—	—	—	—
	LS	—	6.7	6.7	3.3	3.3	—	3.3	—	—	26.7	6.7	—	—	—	—	3.3
	LF	—	30.0	16.7	10.0	—	—	10.0	—	3.3	36.7	6.7	—	—	—	—	—
	Total	—	21.1	10.0	7.8	2.2	1.1	5.6	2.2	1.1	,28.9	6.7	—	—	—	—	1.1

Cont'd...

Cont'd...

Hand-Made and Tailor-Made	LA	—	—	—	—	—	—	—	—	—	—	—	—	—	—	—	—
	LS	—	—	—	—	—	—	—	—	—	—	—	—	—	—	—	—
	LF	—	—	—	—	—	—	—	—	—	—	—	—	—	—	—	—
	Total	—	—	—	—	—	—	—	—	—	—	—	—	—	—	—	—
NR	LA	—	—	—	—	—	—	—	—	—	—	—	—	—	—	—	—
	LS	—	—	—	—	—	—	—	—	—	—	—	—	—	—	—	—
	LF	3.3	—	—	—	—	—	—	—	—	—	—	—	—	—	—	—
	Total	1.1	—	—	—	—	—	—	—	—	—	—	—	—	—	—	—
NA	LA	13.3	13.3	16.7	86.7	96.7	96.7	76.7	86.7	10.0	10.0	10.0	93.3	100.0	100.0	76.7	93.3
	LS	3.3	6.7	10.0	73.3	93.3	96.7	50.0	100.0	6.7	3.3	6.7	86.7	86.7	93.3	73.3	93.3
	LF	—	—	—	80.0	93.3	100.0	63.3	100.0	6.7	6.7	6.7	100.0	100.0	100.0	90.0	100.0

Table shows multiple Responses
A: Saree, B: Saree-Blouse, C: Saree-Petticoat, D: Salwar-Kameez, E: Dress, F: Trouser and Top, G: Gown, H: Any other
NR—No Response
NA—Not Applicable

Verbatim

- "I like to wear synthetic fabric, as they are light in weight, easy to manage and flatter the figure also".
- "I wear what is available to me. I do not ask for new clothes".
- "I wear only white, with a little border may be or self print and preferably cotton, as I am a widow".
- "Due to my age and medical problems, I do not go out anywhere, nor do I need many clothes".

The clothing preference of young-old and old-old has been shown in Table 7, and which has been discussed as under:

Saree: Maximum number of respondents preferred ready-made sarees in both the group. No large variation between two groups was observed. More number of respondents in the younger group (11%) as compared to the older group (2.2%) preferred handloom sarees. In the younger the maximum responses was obtained from respondents who lived with spouse (16.7%), followed by respondents who lived with family (10%) and lastly respondents who lived alone (6.7%). In the older group, an equal number of respondents were found each in the categories of living with spouses and living with family.

Blouse: maximum number of respondents preferred tailor-made blouses, followed by a combination of ready-made and tailor-made.

- More number of respondents in the younger group preferred tailor-made blouse as compared to older group. In the younger group, it was seen more in respondents who lived alone. While in the older group it was seen more in respondents who lived alone, than other two categories.
- A combination of ready-made and tailor-made blouse was seen more in the older group. This was observe more in the respondents who lived with family, followed by respondents living with spouse and respondents living alone, with very marginal difference between the two in the older group. In the younger group, it was seen more in respondents who lived alone and lived with family as compared to respondents with spouse.
- About 16.7 per cent respondents who lived with spouse in younger group and 6.7 per cent respondents who lived with spouse and 3.3 per cent respondents each in the category of living alone and living with family in older group preferred hand-made blouses.

- Merely 3.3 per cent respondents who lived alone in the younger group and 6.7 per cent respondents who lived with spouse in the older group preferred ready-made blouses.

Petticoat: Preference for petticoats was ready-made by most of the respondents followed by tailor-made.

- In ready-made petticoats no major difference between age groups was seen. In the younger group, this was seen more in respondents who lived alone, followed by respondents who lived with family and lastly respondents who lived with spouse. In the older group, it was equally seen in respondents who lived with family and lived with spouse, followed by respondents who lived alone.
- In equal number of respondents in each group (22.2% respectively) prefer tailor-made petticoats. 23.3 per cent respondents each who lived with family in both groups preferred tailor-made petticoat. In the younger group, 26.7 per cent respondents who lived with spouse and 16.7 per cent respondents who lived alone and in older group, 16.7 per cent respondents who lived with spouse and 26.7 per cent respondents who lived alone also preferred the same.
- Barely 10 per cent respondents in the younger group preferred a combination of ready-made and tailor-made petticoat, while only 6.7 per cent of the older group prefer so. In the younger group, this preference was seen maximum in respondents who lived with spouse and living alone. In the older group, no difference was observed between the three living arrangement categories.
- A small percentage of respondents in both groups preferred self-made petticoats. In the younger group, it was seen more in respondents who lived with spouse. (13.3%), followed by 3.03 per cent respondents who lived with family. In older group, 6.7 per cent respondents were equally in both categories—living alone and living with spouse were present.

Salwar-kameez: More number of respondents preferred tailor-made salwar-kameez, out of which an equal number of respondents preferred tailor-made and a combination of ready-made and tailor-made salwar-kameez.

- In the younger group 7.8 per cent respondents preferred tailor-made salwar-kameez, in which 13.3 per cent respondents lived with spouse, followed by 6.7 per cent respondents who lived alone and lastly respondents who lived with family. In the older group, 3.3 per cent respondents who lived alone and 6.7 per cent respondents who lived with spouse also preferred tailor-made salwar-kameez.

- Ready-made salwar-kameez was preferred by 5.6 per cent respondents in younger group as compared to only 3.3 per cent in the older group. More number of respondents was found in the respondents who lived with spouse, followed by respondents who lived with family in the younger group. In the older group, 3.3 per cent respondents who lived alone were present only.
- A combination of hand-made and tailor-made salwar-kameez was preferred by an equal number of respondents in living alone and living with family respondents (10% respectively) and only 3.3 per cent respondents who lived alone, in the younger group (7.8%).
- Hardly 3.3 per cent respondents who lived with spouse in the older group preferred hand-made/self-made salwar-kameez.

Dress: A very small percentage of respondents wore dress and no preference was found between hand-made, tailor-made, ready-made or ready-made and tailor-made between the two groups. 3.3 per cent respondents who lived with spouse in older group preferred hand-made dress, while an equal number of respondents in younger group who lived with family preferred tailor-made dresses. A same percentage of respondents in older group who lived with spouse also referred tailor-made dresses.

- Just 3.3 per cent respondents each in the category of living with spouse and living with family respectively in younger group prefer ready-made dresses.
- A combination of ready-made and tailor-made dresses was preferred by respondents who lived alone and lived with spouse in younger group.

Trouser and Top: Again very few respondents preferred to wear trouser-top and so no preference could be found.

- In the younger group 3.3 per cent respondents who lived with spouse preferred ready-made trouser and tops, while an equal number of respondents who lived alone preferred a combination of ready-made and tailor-made trouser and top.
- In the older group, 6.7 per cent respondents who lived with spouse preferred hand-made garments.

Gown: Maximum number of respondents prefer ready-made gown, followed by tailor-made.

- More number of respondents in younger group preferred ready-made gown, in which maximum respondents were those living with spouse followed by respondents living with family and lastly respondents living alone. In the older group, an equal number of respondents who lived alone and lived with spouse respectively, followed by respondents living with family are there.
- Major difference between the two groups who preferred tailor-made gown was present. With respect to living arrangement in the younger group, maximum response is found in respondents living with spouse, followed by equal number of respondents in other two categories.
- In the older group an equal number of respondents who lived alone and lived with spouse (6.7% respectively) was followed by respondents who lived with family.
- In the younger group, 5.6 per cent respondents preferred a combination of ready-made and tailor-made gown in which more number of respondents was from living with family, followed by equal number of respondents who lived alone and lived with family, followed by equal number of respondents who lived alone and lived with spouse.
- In the older group, 3.3 per cent respondents who lived with spouse preferred hand-made gowns.

Other garments: No preference were found between the groups where garments preferred were tailor-made, ready-made and a combination of ready-made and tailor-made.

- In tailor-made other garments, in the younger group, they were preferred by respondents who lived alone (6.7%), followed by 3.3 per cent respondents who lived with spouse.
- 6.7 per cent in younger group and 3.3 per cent in older group, who lived alone, preferred ready-made garments.
- A combination of ready-made and tailor-made was preferred by 6.7 per cent respondents who lived alone in younger group and 3.3 per cent respondents who lived with spouse in older group.
- Table 8 reveals that the maintenance of garments was carried out by majority with the help of a maid followed by almost equal percentage of respondents who do it by self or with the help of a washing machine.

Table 8 *Maintenance of Garments*

Pattern	*Garments Living Arrange*	*Young-Old*								*Old-Old*							
		A	*B*	*C*	*D*	*E*	*F*	*G*	*H*	*A*	*B*	*C*	*D*	*E*	*F*	*G*	*H*
Maid	LA	50.0	50.0	46.7	13.3	3.3	—	13.3	10.0	66.7	66.7	66.7	3.3	—	—	16.7	6.7
	LS	36.7	40.0	40.0	13.3	3.3	—	20.0	—	53.3	50.0	50.0	3.3	3.3	3.3	16.7	3.3
	LF	33.3	40.0	43.3	—	3.3	—	26.7	—	83.3	70.0	73.3	—	—	3.3	16.7	—
	Total	40.0	43.3	43.3	8.9	3.3	—	20.0	3.3	67.8	62.2	63.3	2.2	1.1	2.2	16.7	3.3
Self	LA	30.0	30.0	30.0	3.3	—	—	3.3	3.3	20.0	20.0	20.0	3.3	—	—	6.7	—
	LS	23.3	23.3	16.7	3.3	—	—	6.7	—	23.3	33.3	26.7	3.3	3.3	3.3	10.0	3.3
	LF	16.7	13.3	13.3	—	—	3.3	—	—	10.0	10.0	6.7	—	—	—	—	—
	Total	23.3	22.2	20.0	2.2	—	1.1	3.3	1.1	17.8	21.1	17.8	2.2	1.1	1.1	5.6	1.1
Washing Machine	LA	6.7	3.3	3.3	3.3	3.3	—	—	—	—	—	—	—	—	—	—	3.3
	LS	30.0	26.7	30.0	—	—	3.3	3.3	—	20.0	13.3	20.0	6.7	—	—	10.0	—
	LF	26.7	26.7	26.7	10.0	—	—	3.3	3.3	10.0	13.3	13.3	3.3	—	—	3.3	—
	Total	21.1	18.9	20.0	4.4	1.1	1.1	2.2	1.1	10.0	8.9	11.1	3.3	—	—	4.4	1.1
Self and Maid	LA	—	—	—	—	—	—	—	—	3.3	3.3	3.3	—	—	—	—	—
	LS	10.0	6.7	3.3	—	—	—	—	—	—	—	—	3.3	—	—	—	—
	LF	16.7	10.0	6.7	3.3	—	—	6.7	—	—	—	—	—	—	—	—	—
	Total	8.9	5.6	3.3	1.1	—	—	2.2	—	1.1	1.1	1.1	1.1	—	—	—	—

Cont'd...

Cont'd...

		A	*B*	*C*	*D*	*E*	*F*	*G*	*H*	*A*	*B*	*C*	*D*	*E*	*F*	*G*	*H*
Washing Machine and Maid	LA	6.7	10.0	6.7	3.3	—	—	3.3	—	—	—	—	—	—	—	—	—
	LS	26.7	23.3	23.3	10.0	6.7	—	20.0	—	—	—	—	—	—	—	—	—
	LF	13.3	6.7	6.7	10.0	—	—	6.7	—	—	6.7	3.3	—	—	—	—	—
	Total	15.6	13.3	12.2	7.8	2.2	—	10.0	—	—	2.2	1.1	—	—	—	—	—
Laundry and Over-lapping	LA	6.7	3.3	—	3.3	—	—	—	—	—	—	—	—	—	—	—	—
	LS	10.0	3.3	3.3	3.3	3.3	—	3.3	—	3.3	—	—	—	—	—	—	—
	LF	23.3	10.0	3.3	—	—	—	3.3	—	—	—	—	—	—	—	—	—
	Total	13.3	5.6	2.2	2.2	1.1	—	2.2	—	1.1	—	—	—	—	—	—	—
NA	LA	13.3	13.3	20.0	83.3	96.7	100.0	80.0	86.7	10.0	10.0	10.0	93.3	100.0	100.0	76.7	90.0
	LS	3.3	3.3	3.3	73.3	90.0	96.7	50.0	100.0	3.3	3.3	3.3	83.3	93.3	93.3	63.3	93.3
	LF	—	6.7	3.3	76.7	96.7	96.7	60.0	96.7	3.3	6.7	6.7	96.7	100.0	96.7	83.3	100.0
	Total	5.6	7.8	8.9	77.8	94.4	97.8	63.3	94.4	5.6	6.7	6.7	91.1	97.8	96.7	74.4	94.4

A: Saree, B: Saree-Blouse, C: Saree-Petticoat, D: Salwar-Kameez, E: Dress, F: Trouser and Top, G: Gown, H: Any other, NA: Not Applicable.
NR: No Response
* Multiple Responses
NA: No specification + respondents not wearing the particular garments.

- A combination of washing machine and maid was seen in more number of respondents, followed by a combination of laundry and overlapping practices. The combination of self and maid was smaller as compared to the other combinations.
- With respect to age groups it was seen that more number of respondents in the older group washed clothes with the help of a maid, than younger group, expect for washing of gowns. Where as more number of respondents were there in the younger group.
- Self-washing was carried out by more number of younger respondents. Washing machine was used more by younger respondents.
- A combination of washing machine and maid was seen more in the younger group and also the practices of laundry and overlapping practice was followed.
- Combination of self maid was also seen more in younger respondents.

Table 9A *Problems in Taking Care of Clothing*

Reasons	*Garments*	*Young-Old*				*Old-Old*			*Total*
		Living Arrangements							
		LA	*LS*	*LF*	*Total*	*LA*	*LS*	*LF*	
Is taking care of clothes a problem?	Yes	6.7	6.7	10.0	7.8	—	—	3.3	1.1
	No	93.3	93.3	90.0	92.2	100.0	100.0	93.3	97.8
	NR	—	—	—	—	—	—	3.3	1.1

Table 9B *Problems Occurred in Taking Care of Clothes*

Reasons	*Young-Old*				*Old-Old*			
	LA	*LS*	*LF*	*Total*	*LA*	*LS*	*LF*	*Total*
Starch and ironing of cotton, cumbersome	—	6.7	—	2.2	—	—	—	—
Leaking of colour in cotton garments	6.7	—	—	2.2	—	—	—	—
Use of naphthalene balls	3.3	—	3.3	2.2	—	—	—	—
Have to take care myself as do not like servant's work	—	—	—	—	—	—	3.3	1.1
NA	90.0	93.3	96.7	93.3	100.0	100.0	96.7	98.9

As seen from Tables 9A and 9B maximum number of respondents did not find taking care of clothes a problem. A small percentage of respondents (4.45%) find taking care of clothes problematic, in which respondents of the younger group are more in number. The reasons given for finding taking care of clothes a problem is many.

- Merely 6.7 per cent respondents who lived with spouse in younger group find applying starch and ironing of cotton clothes cumbersome. "I find applying starch and then ironing quite a task, so I do not prefer to wear cotton clothes frequently".
- Only 6.7 per cent respondents who lived alone in younger group found bleaching of colours as problematic. "Bright colours like peacock blue, indigo, red, dark green bleeding colours, especially if the material is cotton. These clothes were then washed and dried separately, leading to a lot of work".
- Just 3.3 per cent respondents each in the categories of living alone and living with family, in the younger group found use of naphthalene balls for storing clothes cumbersome.
- Merely 3.3 per cent respondents who lived with family, did not like work done by servants, in older group. "I do not like the work/washing done by servants. They do not take proper care while washing nor remove the detergent properly. So, I do my own washing and maintenance."

As revealed by Table 10, it was seen that the major shopping was carried out with a companion, irrespective of the garment. This was followed by self-shopping and recurring of gifts. A large number of respondents have reported that they do not shop. Overlapping practices were the smallest as compared to the other practices.

- With respect to age group, it was seen that there was no major difference between the two age groups regarding shopping with a companion.
- Self-shopping was seen more in younger group.
- No major difference was seen in two groups with respect to receiving gifts. It was seen that more number of respondents in the older group received gifts of blouse/blouse pieces and saree-petticoat.
- No major difference was noticed between the groups with respect to no shopping.

Table 10 *Shopping Practices*

Pattern	Garments Living Arrange	Young-Old								Old-Old							
		A	*B*	*C*	*D*	*E*	*F*	*G*	*H*	*A*	*B*	*C*	*D*	*E*	*F*	*G*	*H*
Self	LA	16.7	20.0	20.0	6.7	3.3	3.3	6.7	—	13.3	16.7	16.7	—	—	—	3.3	—
	LS	43.3	46.7	46.7	16.7	—	3.3	20.0	—	16.7	16.7	16.7	10.0-	—	—	13.3	—
	LF	30.0	23.3	23.3	10.0	—	—	13.3	3.3	20.0	23.3	23.3	3.3	—	—	—	3.3
	Total	30.0	30.0	30.0	11.1	1.1	2.2	13.3	1.1	16.7	18.9	18.9	6.7	—	—	5.6	1.1
With a companion	LA	50.0	46.7	50.0	3.3	—	—	6.7	10.0	43.3	36.7	36.7	—	—	—	3.3	3.3
	LS	60.0	36.7	36.7	13.3	6.7	3.3	16.7	—	56.7	56.7	56.7	—	—	—	6.7	—
	LF	70.0	53.3	50.0	13.3	—	3.3	30.0	—	66.7	66.7	66.7	2.2	—	—	10.0	—
	Total	60.0	45.6	45.6	10.0	2.2	2.2	17.8	3.3	55.6	53.3	53.3	—	—	—	6.7	1.1
Receive gifts	LA	23.3	10.0	10.0	6.7	3.3	3.3	6.7	—	20.0	10.0	10.0	10.0	—	—	—	3.3
	LS	26.7	6.7	6.7	—	—	—	—	—	33.3	23.3	20.0	—	—	—	10.0	—
	LF	33.3	6.7	6.7	—		6.7	3.3	—	30.0	16.7	16.7	3.3	—	—	—	—
	Total	27.8	7.8	7.8	2.2	1.1	3.3	3.3	—	27.8	16.7	15.6	—	—	—	3.3	1.1
Overlapping practice	LA	—	—	—	—	—	—	—	—	3.3	3.3	3.3	—	—	—	—	—
	LS	3.3	—	—	—	—	—	—	—	—	3.3	3.3	—	—	—	—	—
	LF	3.3	3.3	3.3	—	—	3.3	—	—	3.3	—	—	—	—	—	—	—
	Total	2.2	1.1	1.1	—	—	1.1	—	—	2.2	2.2	2.2	—	—	—	—	—

Cont'd...

Cont'd...

		A	*B*	*C*	*D*	*E*	*F*	*G*	*H*	*A*	*B*	*C*	*D*	*E*	*F*	*G*	*H*
No shopping	LA	20.0	20.0	20.0	—	—	—	3.3	3.3	16.7	20.0	16.7	3.3	3.3	3.3	3.3	3.3
	LS	3.3	6.7	6.7	3.3	—	—	3.3	—	13.3	10.0	10.0	—	—	—	3.3	—
	LF	6.7	6.7	6.7	—	—	—	3.3	—	—	—	—	—	—	—	—	—
	Total	10.0	11.1	11.1	1.1	—	—	3.3	1.1	10.0	10.0	8.9	1.1	1.1	1.1	2.2	1.1
NA	LA	13.3	20.0	16.7	86.7	96.7	96.7	83.3	86.7	10.0	16.7	20.0	90.0	96.7	96.7	90.0	90.0
	LS	6.7	16.7	16.7	70.0	93.3	93.3	63.3	100.0	3.3	3.3	6.7	86.7	100.0	100.0	76.7	100.0
	LF	—	20.0	23.3	80.0	100.0	93.3	56.7	96.7	6.7	10.0	10.0	100.0	100.0	100.0	90.0	96.7
	Total	6.7	18.9	18.9	78.9	96.7	94.4	67.8	94.4	6.7	10.0	12.2	92.2	98.9	98.9	85.6	95.6

A: Saree, B: Blouse, C: Saree-Petticoat, D: Salwar-Kameez, E: Dress, F: Trouser and Top, G: Gown, H: Any other, NA: Not Applicable, NR: No Response

* Multiple Responses.

Table 11A *Use of Undergarments*

Use of Undergar-ments	*Young-Old*				*Old-Old*				*Total N*
	Living Arrangemgnes								
	LA	*LS*	*LF*	*Total*	*LA*	*LS*	*LF*	*Total*	
Yes	73.3	76.7	80.0	76.7	43.3	56.7	30.0	43.3	60.0
No	26.7	23.3	20.0	23.3	56.7	43.3			
	70.0	56.7	40.0						

Table 11B *Reasons for not Wearing Undergarments*

Reasons	*Young-Old*				*Old-Old*				*Total N*
	LA	*LS*	*LF*	*Total*	*LA*	*LS*	*LF*	*Total*	
Don't feel the need with age	3.3	10.0	6.7	6.7	3.3	6.7	20.0	10.0	8.35
Skin problems	—	3.3	3.3	2.2	—	—	6.7	2.2	2.2
Don't feel like wearing	—	—	3.3	1.1	—	3.3	6.7	3.3	2.2
Don't feel comfortable	20.0	6.7	6.7	11.1	50.0	30.0	43.3	41.1	26.1
Wear only brassieres	—	3.3	6.7	3.3	—	3.3	—	1.1	2.2
Wear only for outings	—	3.3	—	1.1	3.3	3.3	—	2.2	1.65
Medical problems	3.3	—	—	1.1	6.7	—	3.3	3.3	2.2

It is visible from Tables 11A and 11B that about 60 per cent of the respondents wore undergarments (UG) in which the majority of them fall in the younger group (76.7%), while only 43.3 per cent respondents in the older group wore undergarments. With respect to living arrangement, in the younger group maximum response was from respondents who lived with family, (80%), followed by respondents living with spouse (76.7%) and lastly respondents living alone (73.3%). In the older group, maximum respondents were those who lived with spouse (56.7%), followed by respondents living alone (43.3%) and lastly respondents living with family (30%).

- Nearly 40 per cent of respondents did not wear undergarments regularly. It was observed that more number of older respondents (56,7%) did not use undergarments. In younger respondents only 23.3 per cent did not use undergarments.

With respect to living arrangements, in the older group more number of respondents who lived with family (70%) did not use undergarments, compared with respondents living alone (56.7%) and respondents living with spouse (43.3%). In the younger group, more respondents fall in the living alone (26.7%) category, followed by respondents living with spouse (23.3%) and lastly respondents living alone (20%).

The reasons for not using UG were varied. 26 per cent respondents gave the reason for not wearing UG as they do not feel comfortable, which could be due to a variety of reasons like do not feel the need to wear UG with increasing age, have some skin problems, like itching, rashes, etc.

Some Respondents do not Feel Like Wearing UG

- As one respondents put it "No I do not wear UG, as now I do not feel the need. My menses has stopped, so why wear UG".
- Another said, "If I were UG, It starts itching and I develop rashes. Also, with the increase in age", I do not feel the need to wear UG.
- Some respondents wear only brassieres, while some others wear UG, if they have to go out for some outings only.
- A small per cent of respondents gave the reason as medical problems for not wearing UG.

Table 12A *Particularness Regarding Your Clothes?*

Age Group	*Young-Old*				*Old-Old*				*Total N*
	Living Arrangement								
	LA	*LS*	*LF*	*Total*	*LA*	*LS*	*LF*	*Total*	
I was always particular and still am	43.3	60.0	46.7	50.0	43.3	50.0	40.0	44.4	47.2
I was particular before, now I am not	13.3	30.0	13.3	13.3	46.7	6.7	33.3	18.9	18.9
I was not particular before and even now I am not	43.3	10.0	40.0	40.0	40.0	43.3	26.7	36.7	33.9

Table 12B *Comments Made Regarding Particularness About Clothes*

Age Group	*Young-Old*				*Old-Old*			*Total*
	Living Arrangement							
	LA	*LS*	*LF*	*Total*	*LA*	*LS*	*LF*	
Economic condition was not too good before, so less number of sarees earlier	—	—	3.3	1.1	—	—	—	—
Does not like applying starch to clothes	—	3.3	3.3	2.2	—	—	—	—
Convenience matters most	3.3	3.3	—	2.2	—	—	—	—
Always wear starched clothes	—	—	6.7	2.2	—	—	—	—
Have medical problems so difficult to maintain	—	—	—	—	—	—	3.3	1.1
After spouse death lost interest in clothes	—	—	—	—	3.3	—	—	1.1
NA	96.7	93.3	90.0	93.3	96.7	100.0	96.7	97.8

Table shows multiple responses.
NA = Respondents who were particular/who did not.

- It can be seen from Table 12A that about 47.2 per cent of respondents were always particular about their clothes and still are seen more in the younger group (50%), than older group (44.4%). This tendency was found more in respondents who lived with spouse in both the groups (60% YO and 50% OO). In the younger group, it was followed by respondents who lived with family (46.7%) and respondents who lived with alone (43.3%). In the older group, it was followed by respondents who lived alone (43.3%) and respondents who lived with family (40%).
- Nearly 33.9 per cent respondents were not particular about their clothes before, i.e., before attaining 60 years of age and they still were not particular. This tendency was seen more in older group (36.7%) as compared to younger group (31.1%). In the older group, it was seen more in respondents who lived with spouse

(43.3%), followed by respondents who lived alone (40%) and lastly respondents living with family (26.7%). In the younger group, it was seen more in respondents who lived alone (43.3%), followed by respondents who lived with family (40%) and lastly respondents who lived with spouse (10%).

- Only 18.9 per cent respondents were more particular about the clothes they wore before attaining 60 years age of age or in their youth and at present they are not so particular as before, which is seen in equal number of respondents in both the groups. In the younger group it was seen in more number in respondents who lived alone (43.3%), followed by respondents living with family (40%) and lastly respondents living with spouse (10%). In the older group, it was seen more in respondents who lived with spouse (43.3%), followed by respondents living alone (40%) and lastly respondents who lived with family.

Comments Made Regarding Particularness about Clothes

These have been shown in Table 12B. The reasons for not being particular about the clothes were varied.

- One respondent put it, "When I was young, the economic condition of the family was not good. So, I had very few sarees, e.g., like a few good sarees for wearing outside and three-four not so good sarees for wearing in the house".
- A few respondents did not like applying starch to their clothes, so they found that cotton would crumple very easily.
- A few busy women pointed that convenience mattered most to them, so they wore whatever was convenient and easily manageable.
- A few respondents as against the above/earlier one's, said that they wore only starched clothes.
- One respondent said, "I lost interest in clothes after my husband's death. Earlier I used to get ready, wear make-up jewellery and do everything available. Everyone used to appreciate the efforts I took while dressing up. But, now after husband's death, I feel very lonely and feel what is the need to get ready and for whom should I do it? There is one to appreciate anything".

Table 13A *Physical Change Encountered with Growing Age*

Age Group	*Young-Old*				*Old-Old*			*Total*
	Living Arrangements							
	LA	*LH*	*LF*	*Total*	*LA*	*LH*	*LF*	
Physical Changes								
Increase in weight	16.7	30.0	40.0	28.9	16.7	13.3	16.7	15.6
Decrease in weight	26.7	30.0	26.7	27.8	23.3	36.7	30.0	30.0
Dry skin/Formation of wrinkles	30.0	6.7	6.7	14.4	36.7	20.0	36.7	31.1
Muscle tone is lost	6.7	6.7	6.7	6.7	3.3	10.0	6.7	6.7
Swiftness/agility decreased	—	23.3	16.7	13.3	6.7	16.7	6.7	10.0
Menopausal change	—	6.7	3.3	3.3	—	—	3.3	1.1
Hearing and vision problem	3.3	—	3.3	2.2	3.3	—	6.7	3.3
Grey hair	—	—	—	—	3.3	3.3	—	2.2
Knee problem	10.0	10.0	3.3	7.8	6.7	6.7	3.3	5.6
Medical reason/Accident/Multiple fracture	10.0	—	6.7	5.6	3.3	6.7	—	3.3
Problems while sitting down/getting up	—	—	6.7	2.2	6.7	—	3.3	3.3
Discomfort while wearing saree	3.3	—	—	1.1	—	—	—	—
Sleeplessness, loss of appetite	3.3	—	3.3	2.2	3.3	—	—	1.1
Need constant rest	36.7	20.0	3.3	20.0	23.3	23.3	30.0	25.6
No relevant change	13.3	3.3	20.0	12.2	30.0	16.7	23.3	23.3
NA	6.7	16.7	20.0	14.4	3.3	16.7	16.7	12.2

* Multiple responses, so total might not add upto 100 per cent.

The physical change encountered with growing age has been presented in Table 13A and has been discussed as under:

- The major physical changes encountered with growing age were increase or decrease in weight, dryness of skin, formation of wrinkles, decrease in agility and the need for constant rest. These changes were found in almost equal percentage in both the group's, i.e., younger and older groups.
- The other changes observed by the respondent were loss of muscle tone, knee problems, other medical reasons/problems like multiple fractures, frequent small accidents, and problems

occurred while sitting down or getting up, sleeplessness, loss of appetite. A few other problems were hearing and vision problems, grey hair, discomfort due to wearing a saree.

- A few respondents found no relevant change.

Table 13B *Problems while Dressing Due to Physical Change*

Age Group	*Young-Old*				*Old-Old*			*Total*
	Living Arrangements							
	LA	*LH*	*LF*	*Total*	*LA*	*LH*	*LF*	
Physical Changes								
Do not feel like wearing thick sarees	—	—	3.3	1.1	—	—	—	—
Do not like to wear sarees, with rising age	—	—	3.3	1.1	10.0	—	—	3.3
Would prefer salwar/kameez/gown	—	—	3.3	1.1	6.7	—	—	2.2
Wore gown/salwar-kameez, not preferred, so switched to sarees again	—	—	—	—	3.3	—	—	1.1
Can't sit on floor	3.3	—	—	1.1	—	—	3.3	1.1
Need help to wear clothes	3.3	3.3	3.3	3.3	—	—	3.3	1.1
Blouses are loose	—	—	—	—	—	—	3.3	1.1
Takes more time to dress up	—	—	—	—	3.3	—	—	1.1
Back pain, hinders wearing clothes comfortably	3.3	—	—	1.1	3.3	—	3.3	2.2
Wear clothes as it is a social necessity	3.3	—	—	1.1	—	—	—	—
Cannot wear tight fitting clothes	—	6.7	—	2.2	6.7	—	13.3	6.7
Cannot wear synthetic fabric	—	3.3	—	1.1	—	—	6.7	2.2
Accessories reduced with age	3.3	—	—	1.1	—	—	—	—
Skin problems	3.3	3.3	—	2.2	—	3.3	—	1.1
NA	180.0	180.0	190.0	183.3	170.0	196.7	1,667	177.8

Table 13B shows that the problems encountered while dressing due to physical changes were varied right from difficulty in wearing and handling sarees, physical discomfort to back problems, wearing clothes as a social necessity and reduction in accessories.

- A large number of respondents said that they did like to wear sarees due to age, as it reduces or hinders mobility, also thick sarees, due to their weight are not preferred. A few respondents would prefer to wear salwar-kameez or gown instead of a saree, but are not used to it/not comfortable.

As one respondent in older group puts it, "Due to some health problems, I started wearing gowns and salwar-kameez, but I could not feel comfortable in it, as I was not used to wearing such garments. So, I switched over to wearing sarees again and now manage sarees properly along with the health problems".

- With decrease in muscle tone, a few respondents found that blouse become loose and it takes them a lot of time to dress-up now as compared to when they were young. Also, due to decreased musculature and agility it becomes problematic to sit down or wear clothes comfortably. Some cannot tolerate tight fitting clothes and would prefer loose, soft clothing.
- Tolerance to wear synthetic fabrics also was reduced.
- Some respondents found that due to clothes skin problems were occurring.
- Accessories were reduced by the younger group.
- One respondents in the younger group said that, "To tell you the truth, I hate wearing clothes; I wear clothes as it is social necessity and if I do not wear clothes people will ostracize me from the society".

The changes suggested for comfortable clothing has been presented in Table 14 and these have been discussed as follows:

The major suggestion given by the respondents for comfortable clothing were that clothes should be comfortable and easily maintained and one should wear clothes in accordance to one's age and culture.

- No major difference was observed between the age groups for the suggestion that clothes should be comfortable and easily maintained. More number of respondents were observed in the younger group for the living alone (40% YO, 30% OO) and living with spouse category (36.7% YO and 26.7% OO) category. While more respondents were there in the older group for the living with family category (46.7% OO, 30% YO).

Table 14 *Changes Suggested for Comfortable Clothing*

Age of Respondent	*Young-Old*				*Old-Old*			*Total*
	Living Arrangements							
	LA	*LS*	*LF*	*Total*	*LA*	*LS*	*LF*	
Physical Changes								
Wear clothes according to age	26.7	23.3	20.0	23.3	23.3	36.7	46.7	35.6
Clothes should be comfortable and easily maintained	40.0	36.7	30.0	35.6	30.0	26.7	46.7	34.4
Wear clothes according to one's wish	10.0	6.7	6.7	7.8	—	3.3	6.7	3.3
Should wear simple cotton clothes	3.3	6.7	10.0	6.7	—	—	3.3	1.1
Clothes should cover the whole body	—	16.7	3.3	6.7	13.3	3.3	—	5.6
Sarees should be soft and light in weight	13.3	13.3	10.0	12.2	3.3	3.3	—	2.2
Wear clothes according to own culture	6.7	10.0	10.0	8.9	13.3	6.7	3.3	7.8
Do not wear synthetic fibre	3.3	3.3	—	2.2	—	3.3	—	1.1
Avoid bright colours	10.0	6.7	—	5.6	—	3.3	3.3	2.2
Clothes should be easy to wear	3.3	6.7	13.3	7.8	3.3	3.3	10.0	5.6
Salwar-kameez/gown comfortable	3.3	10.0	13.3	8.9	—	6.7	6.7	4.4
Stitched sarees should be available	—	3.3	—	1.1	—	—	—	—
Cotton blouse pieces are unavailable	—	10.0	—	3.3	—	—	—	—
No change, our sarees are good	3.3	—	10.0	4.4	—	—	3.3	1.1
No changes suggested	33.3	16.7	13.3	21.1	46.7	36.7	20.0	34.4

- More number of older group respondents said that one should wear clothes according to their age. Major difference was found in the respondents who live with family, where more number of respondents were there in older group (46.7% OO, 20% YO). This was also observed in the living with spouse category, where 36.7 per cent respondents were in older group, while only 23.3 per cent respondents were in the younger group.

- Major difference between the younger and older group was not observed for the suggestion that clothes should reflect our culture. A difference was observed between the living alone category, where older respondents (13.3%) were more than younger (6.7%). In the other 2 categories the younger respondents were more, living with spouse 10 per cent YO and 6.7 per cent OO and living with family 10 per cent YO and 3.3 per cent OO.
- More number of respondents in the younger group said that the sarees should be soft and light in weight (12.2% YO and 2.2% OO). Respondents living alone were more in the younger group (13.3% YO), than older group (3.3%). This was also true for the respondents living with spouse. 10 per cent respondents who lived with family were present in the younger group only.
- Avoidance of bright colours was seen more in younger group which have respondents who lived alone (10%) and respondents who lived with spouse (6.7%). In the older group respondents were there in equal number in the categories respondents living with spouse and living with family respectively.
- Clothes should be easy to wear was again seen more in younger groups, with a very small difference between the two groups (7.8% YO and 5.6% OO). A small difference was seen in the categories of living with spouse (6.7% YO and 3.3% OO) and living with family (13.3% YO and 10% OO). No difference in the category living alone, with 3.3 per cent respectively was seen in both the groups.
- 6.65 per cent respondents felt that salwar-kameez or gown were more comfortable to wear. This was seen in more number of respondents in younger group (8.9% YO 4.4% OO). Difference was seen in respondents who lived with spouse (10% YO and 6.7% OO) and respondents living with family (13.3% and YO 6.7% OO). Only 3.3 per cent respondents who lived alone in younger group were there.
- 6.15 per cent respondents said that clothes should cover the whole body, in which a little difference was present between the two groups (6.7% YO and 5.6% OO). In the younger group more number of respondents were present in the respondents who lived with spouse (16.7%), followed by 3.3 per cent respondents who lived with family. In the older group 13.3 per cent respondents lived alone, while 3.3 per cent respondents lived with spouse.

- As one respondent put it, "Clothes should cover the whole body. Nowadays we see a lot of girls wearing skimpy clothes, showing their bellies and what not. It does not look good, nor is it in accordance to our culture".
- In opposition to the above, 5.5 per cent respondents feel that one should wear what one wishes or likes. This is again seen more in the younger group (7.8% YO) than older group (3.3%). More number of respondents are seen in the living alone category (10%) in the younger group, followed by equal number of respondents in the categories living with spouse and living with family respectively. In the older group respondents living with family are more (6.7%) as compared to respondents living with spouse (3.3%).
- More number of respondents in the younger group (6.7%) than older group feel that one should wear simple cotton clothes. This was seen in respondents living with family (10%), followed by respondents living with spouse (6.7%) and lastly respondents living alone (3.3%) in the younger group. 3.3 per cent respondents living with family were present in older group only.
- Only 10 per cent respondents who lived with spouse in the younger group felt that cotton blouse are unavailable. As one respondents said, "Nowadays pure cotton blouses are nor available easily, what is available is a mix of fibres-cotton + synthetic, which I do not like".
- Just 3.3 per cent respondents who lived with spouse in the younger group said that stitched saree's should be available. "Wearing and draping of saree becomes quite cumbersome as you grow old. Instead, if stitched sarees are made available, it would be very easy to wear a saree; one just has to tie the string (Nada)".
- About 27.75 per cent respondents gave no suggestions for comfortable clothing, in which respondents in the older group were more (34.4% OO, 21.1% YO). A difference was seen with respect to living arrangement, where more number of respondents in all living arrangement categories was present in older group.
- Merely 2.75 per cent respondents gave no suggestion as they felt that our sarees are good. This was given more by the younger group (4.4%) than older (1.1%).

Table 15 *Requirement of Shops for Elderly*

Age of Respondent		*Young-Old*				*Old-Old*			
		Living Arrangements							
	Response	*LA*	*LS*	*LF*	*Total*	*LA*	*LS*	*LF*	*Total*
Physical Changes									
Older persons require shops catering to their own needs	Yes (%)	6.7	36.7	10.0	17.8	16.7	23.3	16.7	18.9
	No (%)	90.0	63.3	90.0	81.1	83.3	76.7	83.3	81.1
	NR (%)	3.3	—	—	1.1	—	—	—	—
Heard of special shops catering to elderly needs	Yes (%)	23.3	16.7	13.3	17.8	23.3	26.7	6.7	18.9
	No (%)	76.7	83.3	86.7	82.2	76.7	70.0	93.3	80.0
	NR (%)	—	—	—	—	—	3.3	—	1.1
Thought of special clothes catering to elderly need	Yes (%)	23.3	23.3	20.0	22.2	23.3	23.3	3.3	16.7
	No (%)	76.7	76.7	76.7	76.7	76.7	76.7	96.7	83.3
	NR (%)	—	—	3.3	1.1	—	—	—	—

- As visible from Table 15, almost 81.1 respondents did not think that older persons require shops catering to their own needs. This was felt equally by the respondents in both the groups. Difference was observed in the living arrangements categories, where more number of respondents were present in the younger group. In the categories living alone (90% YO, 83.3% OO) and living with family (90% YO and 83.3% OO). More number of respondents who were living with spouse were present in older group (76.7% OO, 63.3% YO).
- Only 18.35 respondents thought that older persons should have shops catering to their needs. A small difference was seen in the two age groups, (17.8% YO and 18.9% OO). With respect to living arrangement, more number of respondents who lived with family and lived alone were found in older group, while respondents living with spouse were more in younger group.
- Nearly 81.1 per cent respondents had not heard about special shops catering to the elderly needs. There is a small difference between the two groups (82.2% YO and 80% OO). Respondents who lived alone (76.7% YO and OO) were same in both the groups, while respondents who lived with spouse were more in

the younger group (83.3% YO and 70% OO), and respondents who lived with family were more in the older group (93.3% OO and 86.7% YO).

- Only 18.35 per cent respondents had heard of special shops catering to the elderly needs, in which a small difference was seen in both the groups (17.8% YO and 18.9% OO). With respect to living arrangement, no difference was found in respondents who lived alone (23.3% YO and OO). A large difference is seen in respondents living with spouse (16.7% YO and 26.7% OO) and respondents living with family (13,3% YO and 6.7% YO). We have heard about shops which categories specified to older people and their need, abroad, in the USA, but not seen or heard about any such thing in India.
- Almost 80 per cent respondents have thought of special clothes that should be available, catering to the elder's needs. This was seen more in older respondents (83.3% OO) than younger (76.7%). No difference was seen in the living alone (76.7% YO and OO) and living with spouse (76.7% YO and OO) categories. Difference was seen in living with family category, where more respondents are from older group (96.7% OO and 76.7% YO).
- Nearly 19.45 per cent respondents did not feel the need of designer clothes, catering to elderly needs, in which more respondents were from the younger group (22.2%). No difference was seen in the living arrangement categories, living alone (23.3% YO and OO) and living with spouse (23.3% YO and OO). A great difference was seen in the living with family category, where more respondents were there in the younger group (20% YO and 3.3% OO).

Factors Influencing Clothing Patterns

The first six factors which influenced clothing patterns in young-age and old-age, for both the groups, young-old and old-old were the same. They were—culture, society, comfort, economics, climate and religion. The only difference observed is that in young age, culture and society are the first preference, followed by comfort, while in old-age, comfort is the first preference, followed by culture and society at the second and third preferences.

- The 7th preference in young age was fashion, which slips to be the 11th preference in old-age and the 7th preference is health.
- The 8th preference is relatives in both the groups, in young age and old-age.
- The 9th and 10th preference in young age were occupation and friends, while in old age, they were friends and occupation.
- 11th preference in young age was education, while in old age, it was fashion.
- 12th preference in young age was health (which was 7th preference in old age), while in old-age it is education.
- The 13th preference in both the groups was same—dwelling place.
- The 14th preference in both the groups was same—media.
- The 15th preference in both the groups was same—migration.
- 66.7 per cent respondents in young age and 72.3 per cent respondents in old age reported no influence on their clothing pattern.

In conclusion, it can be said, that while culture and society influenced clothing pattern, when the respondents were young, in old-age comfort matter most.

In young age fashion, influenced the clothing pattern (as it is in 7th place), while old-age fashion does not matter (11th preference). In old-age health also matters (7th preference).

Factors Most Influencing Clothing Pattern

- Clothing preference in young age—society, culture, comfort and fashion (also economic, climate, religion)
- Clothing preference in old age—comfort, culture, society and health (also economic, climate, religion)

Factors Least Influencing

- In young age, education, health, dwelling place, media and migration.
- In old age, fashion education, dwelling place, media and migration.

Conclusions

- Most women prefer and wear saree/blouse/petticoat sets.

- Most women, especially those who live with spouse, prefer wearing saree/blouse/petticoat in the day. It was also the most common garment for other activities and occasions like going for walks, meeting friends or on festivals.
- Salwar-kameez and gown were also preferred by women, but more women from the younger group used these.
- Seasonal variation in clothing was very less. For all the reasons, respondents preferred wearing light/pastel coloured, cotton fabrics with small or no prints. A small percentage of women preferred synthetic clothes in monsoons.
- Most women preferred ready-made sarees, petticoats and gowns and tailor-made blouses. No specific pattern or preference emerged for salwar-kameez, dress and trouser-tops.
- Majority of the respondents did not find taking care of clothes problematic.
- Majority of respondents shop with a companion, mostly for saree/blouse/petticoat sets. More young women shop alone.
- About 60 per cent of the respondents, mostly young-old women wear undergarments. Those who did not use under garments felt some discomfort while wearing them.
- Nearly 47.2 per cent of the entire sample felt that they always were and still are particular about their clothes. Most of these women, in both groups, lived with the spouse.
- An equal percentage of young and old women felt that there were physical changes due to age and this led to problems in dressing. Some problems mentioned were:
  - — Difficulty in wearing sarees, especially heavy and thick ones.
  - — Reduction in use of accessories.
  - — Problems in blouse fittings due to loss of muscle tone.
- Most women felt that they should wear clothes that are comfortable, easy to maintain and in accordance to one's age and culture.
- Majority of the respondents did not feel the need to have shops catering to the clothing needs of elderly.
- Comfort and health have become important influencing factors besides culture, society, economics, climate and religion influencing clothing preferences and choices of elderly women.

References

Bond, John, Peter Coleman et al. (1999) *Ageing in Society: An Introduction to Social Gerontology*. Sage Publications, London.

Das, N.P. and U. Shah. (2001) The Social and Health Status of the Elderly in India: Evidence from Recent National Level Date. Department of Statistics, Ministry of Planning, Government of India, New Delhi.

Gowli, R. Geetha, P.J. Reddy and D. Usha Rani. (2003) *Elderly Women: A Study of the Unorganized Sector*. Discovery Publishing House, New Delhi.

Goyal, N. (2000) *A Study on the Clothing Practices, Interest and Needs of the Elderly*. Department of Clothing and Textile, M.S. University of Baroda, Vadodara.

Hurlock, E.B. (1981) *Developmental Psychology: A Life Span Approach*. McGraw Hill Inc., New York.

10

Late Middle Age

A Turning Point for Changes in Lifestyle, Diet, Physical Activity and Disease

VANISHA S. NAMBIAR

Decline in functional abilities or ageing begins long before one reaches age 60. Late middle age (+45 years) is an important period in life during which changes in dietary patterns and lifestyle may occur and they may have an impact on the health of the individuals.

Late middle age is particularly an important period for both men and women, as it is during this period that age-related disorders begin to manifest themselves overtly. It is during this period that preventive approaches involving diet, nutrition and lifestyle changes can have their maximum impact. Late middle age is a time that coincides with reduced demands on physical work due to shrinking family size and onset of hormonal changes in women due to approaching menopause.

Nutrition Transition

Diet and lifestyle factors become increasingly more important to understand and control in order to help an individual lead a healthy life.

A vast majority of the countries in Asia, Latin America, Northern Africa and the Middle East have now experienced 'nutrition transition' whereby diets high in unrefined carbohydrates and fibre are replaced by diets containing a higher proportion of fats, particularly saturated fatty acids and sugars and as a result the proportion of the overweight or obese population is already increasing rapidly (Gopalan, 1992). Gopalan also reported a progressive increase in the intake of edible fat with a preference for hydrogenated fat (in case of middle class) and a high intake of ghee in affluent class.

Socio-demography Diet Lifestyle and Physical Activity Pattern

The urge to rise has driven India's 300 million strong middle aged middle class into a consumer economy that is seeing no bounds. Our paper on relationship between socio-demographic indicators, income, lifestyle and caloric intake in post-menopausal women, reported results on the nutrient intake, nutritional status and physical activity pattern in post-menopausal women (45–58 years) from two income groups in urban Vadodara. The prevalence of overweight/obesity and its relation to income, lifestyle and caloric intake from 150 women belonging to affluent income group (Group A; $n=75$) and middle income group (Group B; $n=75$) was also assessed (Nambiar and Seshadri, 2002).

Income had a significant relationship with the calorie intake and fat intake wherein the affluent group consumed 4 times more fat than the RDA. The energy expenditure pattern showed that the subjects of the affluent Group A, spent significantly more time on sedentary activities compared to Group B subjects who spent more time on moderate activities. Socio-economic characteristics such as ethnic group, family size and food habits had a marked influence on the nutrient intake of the subjects, energy expenditure and anthropometric profile.

Despite a decreased dietary intake of energy and fat with increase in age, the prevalence of overweight/obesity on the basis of Body Mass Index (BMI) was higher in both the groups (Group A–62% and Group B–44%). Our results reveal that the time spend on sedentary activities and consumption of total calories and fat were the main factors positively associated with the overweight/obesity in these subjects, which highlights the need for appropriate interventions and increased awareness about the risks of obesity in this population (Nambiar and Seshadri, 2002). As age advances there was a tendency for the subjects to make changes in their dietary habits. Some of these changes were due to presence of diseases in the subject or in the family. Others were apparently mediated by an increases health consciousness and a desire to avoid excess gain in body weight. Income was not a major factor influencing these changes as both the middle class as well as affluent class reported similar changes in past five years.

NNMB data (http://www.NNMBIndia.org/publications.html) also revealed that as the Indian population moved up the socio-economic ladder, their intake of legumes, vegetables, milk, sugar and sweets increased with substitution of rice and wheat for millets. These changes could result in a reduction in the fibre content of the diet. Such a change in the initial years of development may be beneficial as it results in correction of the energy deficits by improvements in the nutrient quality of the diets. However, with increase in affluence, harmful effects of the dietary change have become obvious.

Dual Burden of Malnutrition in Middle Age

Dual burden of malnutrition is evident in the middle aged population, while overweight and obesity as the consequences of overeating high fat and energy dense foods, there is also evidence that micronutrient deficiencies are very common among middle aged and elderly populations, even in the most developed countries, and they have increasingly been linked to risk of chronic diseases. Among the micronutrient deficiencies, calcium, zinc, folic acid, vitamin B_6, B_{12} and D are common. Sub-clinical vitamin and mineral deficiencies may also contribute to the pathogenesis of declining neuro-cognitive function with age (Tucker and Burnanapin, 2001; Popkin, 1998; Solomons and Anderson, 2002).

Changes in diet and activity patterns are fuelling the obesity epidemic. These rapid changes in the levels and composition of dietary and activity/inactivity patterns in transitional societies are related to a number of socio-economic and demographic changes (Popkin, 2001).

Physical Activity Pattern and Anthropometric Profile

Although reduction in the caloric intake with increasing age is also reported, this reduction in energy intake is not significant to compensate the reduced energy expenditure and there is often a gradual but steady increase in body weight and fat mass through the fifth or sixth decade of life in females. It is the general impression that Indian women regardless of the social class continue to do physical work which may offset the tendency to overweight or obesity in them.

A Decline in Physical Activity Pattern

Middle age is also characterized by a progressive decline in both occupational and leisure time activity which may lead to many metabolic disorders. There is ample evidence that simple-stretching, range-of-motion and deep breathing exercises significantly lowered blood pressure and increased mobility (56–98 years) (Casperson et al., 1991). This study reported that most of the subjects were overweight and had never exercised regularly. All complained of chronic ailments, including arthritis, hypertension, heart diseases and diabetes. Flexibility in hand activities and mobility improved after 6 weeks of exercise as did self-reported bone and joint pain upon performing daily tasks.

A decline in physical activities commonly occurs with ageing which may have its origin in diverse factors. Studies by Durnin (1983) comparing the physical activities of various age groups had indicated that the population above 50 years seemed to have similar degrees of mechanical efficiency as the younger men, but there was a general diminution of neuromuscular coordination, which could be one of the factors resulting in reduced physical activity in the late middle age. He also reported that with grown up children the work of a housewife steadily decreased after 45 years and fell proportionately more than that of a man upto 70 years or so.

A lack in physical exercise may lead to an increase in total body weight which in turn may be associated with the development of many diseases and disorders in the middle aged population. An increased liability to suffer from one or more of the degenerative diseases of the circulatory and respiratory systems and particularly of the bones and joints in the middle aged may restrict their physical activity.

There is substantial evidence in adults that regular physical activities attenuates with overweight or obesity including prevention of diabetes and coronary artery disease risk factors (Blair et al., 1999; Pan et al., 1997; Misra and Khurana, 2008).

Changes in Body Composition

Anthropometry is the most common method for assessing the nutritional status. This method is based on the assumption that deficiencies or excesses of nutrients are associated with deviation in body composition from the normal and that these are reflected in the anthropometric measurements. With advancing age fat mass increases by 5–9 kg and that is a decrease in the fat free mass (FFM) by 2–3 kg due to a reduction of the muscle mass. There is a redistribution of fat, subcutaneous fat being deposited more on the trunk in the elderly than on the limbs, compared to the younger people. There is also a change in the ratio of fat between the subcutaneous and the deeper truncal areas with ageing, more of fat being in the deeper regions in older people. Body composition changes with age and a normal part of ageing is the gradual decrease in muscle mass, and with its strength, known as sacropenia. Changes in dietary patterns, physical activity and lifestyle occurring during late middle age in women, may have an impact on the health of the individuals as they turn into the elderly population.

The double burden of undernutrition and overweight or obesity in an ageing population poses tremendous challenges for developing countries. There a great potential for prevention of these diseases through healthy lifestyles that include physical activity and nutritious diets.

Disease Profile

The role of nutrition as a factor in the causation of chronic diseases, usually age related received a lot of attention, although it is difficult to arrive at a consensus. Several diseases have been identified as age related but the major diseases which have been said to be related to nutrition are the disorders of the bone and chronic diseases like coronary heart disease (CHD), hypertension, diabetes mellitus, obesity and osteoporosis. The pattern of so-called modern diseases makes their appearance in late middle age. These disease, i.e., cardiovascular diseases, diabetes mellitus and osteoporosis are increasingly engaging the attention of the nutritionists.

Dietary Pattern vs Disease Profile

We assessed the dietary patterns and their relation to relationship with the disease profile in postmenopausal women (Nambiar and Seshadri, 2004). A highly significant difference was seen in the intake of pulses, fruits, milk and milk products between the two groups: the total consumption for the affluent group (Group A) being much higher than the subjects of the middle income (Group B) subjects.

The major confirmed chronic degenerative chronic diseases reported were hypertension (34%), osteoarthritis (27%), multiple disorders (CVD, diabetes and blood pressure, 7%), and 59 subjects (39.3%) complained of symptoms which were suggestive of disorders of one or more systems of the body. Of the 150, the per cent of subjects who reported to be healthy having no symptoms of disorders or disease was 31.3 per cent. Forty-five per cent of the subjects from Group A and 33 per cent from Group B had reached menopause. Another 15 per cent of the women were suffering from irregular periods. The mean age for menopause was 46 years. The complaints of these women were mental irregularities, gastric upsets, hot flushes, depression, and diminished stamina, fluctuations in moods, irritability, stiffness and pain in joints, memory lapses and headaches. Our results clearly indicated that, as age advanced there was a tendency for the subjects to make changes in their dietary habits. Some of these changes occurred because of the presence of diseases in the subject or in the family. Others were apparently mediated by an increased health consciousness and a desire to avoid excess gain in body weight (Nambiar and Seshadri, 2004).

These results clearly indicate that there is a strong association between nutrition and many degenerative disorders commonly affecting the ageing. As the population base shifts its mean age upwards, it becomes increasingly important for health care practitioners, managers and planners to understand the dietary and nutrient intake patterns and requirements of the middle aged and age-related health disorders, both of which are closely linked to the socio-economic condition of the population. Available epidemiological data show that the appearance of some of these diseases in middle age is exacerbated by affluence, plentiful supply of foods especially the energy rich ones, excessive consumption of refined foods and relative lack of exercise in the middle age.

Diet and Bone Health with Advancing Age

Progressive loss of bone is a physiological event which accompanies advance age. This occurs both in men and women beginning in the fourth decade of life. However, the bone loss is relatively greater and easier to detect in women in that it begins with the onset of menopause. In one out of four women this loss of bone mineral exceeds physiological limits to become pathological: post-menopausal osteoporosis. This diffuse decalcifying osteopathy is considered to be the most frequent metabolic bone disorder in women characterized by bone pain, fractures and skeletal deformities.

Osteomalacia (adult rickets) is characterized by decreased bone density, primarily due to loss of calcium of the protein matrix, hence bone of abnormal calcium-protein ratio. This decrease results from a lack of vitamin D which is needed by the body to utilize calcium in bone formation. Osteoporosis, on the other hand, is defined as decrease in bone density due to loss of total substance without change in chemical composition. This is the predominant form of bone loss in pre- and post-menopausal women. Problems such as osteoporosis may be aggravated by inadequate intake of one or more nutrients as age advances. Increasing the dietary intake of milk and other foods is a simple way to improve the diet for bone health. Diet may affect the skeletal health throughout the life cycle. Decreased calcium intake is reported to cause a positive shift in calcium balance. It has been established that 1, 25 $(OH)^2$ vitamin D concentrations are decreased in healthy individuals with age. These alterations in vitamin D are associated with a decline in intestinal calcium absorption efficiency. This plus (+) a decreased supply of 1, 25 $(OH)^2$ vitamin D action was suggested as a contributing factor to age-related bone loss and osteoporosis (Heaney, 1986).

Advancing Age and Metabolic Syndrome

Cardiovascular diseases are the leading causes of death and debilitation. Epidemiological studies have reported a positive relationship between increased levels of plasma lipoproteins and coronary heart disease (CHDs). Prevalence of obesity and the metabolic syndrome is rapidly increasing in developing countries, leading to increased morbidity and mortality due to type II diabetes mellitus (T2 DM) and cardiovascular diseases.

Our study (Nambiar and Guin, 2007), aimed to assess the prevalence of hyperglycemia and hyperlipidemia among middle aged and older (37–73 years) population in a university setup. The results revealed that the mean fasting blood glucose (FBG), total cholesterol (TC), high density lipoprotein cholesterol (HDL-C), low density cholesterol (LDL-C) and very low density cholesterol (VLDL-C) and triglycerides (TG) were 100 mg/dl, 200 mg/dl, 42 mg/dl, 125 mg/dl, 33 mg/dl and 166 mg/dl respectively. Out of the 162 subjects studied only 21.6 per cent had normal biochemical parameters, whereas 29 per cent of the subjects were hyperlipidemics. The remaining 50.6 per cent had either a high TC or TG value. Females in general had higher values as well as higher atherogenic indices as compared to the male subjects.

Since the average age for these post-menopausal female subjects was 51 years, wherein the protective effects of estrogen was limited, they were at risk for chronic degenerative disorders (CDDs) and therapeutic lifestyle changes are advised for these subjects. Our study highlighted the fact that CDDs are emerging public health problem even in the highly educated population due to ignorance and negligence in selection of healthy foods. Such a trend is now obvious in most of the developing countries and has invaded the middle aged population of India at an unbridled momentum (Nambiar and Guin, 2007).

Our study on post-menopausal women revealed that the disease profile of the subject's changes markedly as the subjects aged. Income also had an impact on the disease profile of the subjects. When current health disorders were compared with those of past ten years, significant increase was seen in the prevalence of some symptoms, which were mainly related to the oral cavity, GI, respiratory system and central nervous system. In the confirmed chronic diseases, high blood pressure ranked first followed by arthritis, heart problems and diabetes mellitus and a combination of one or more of these (Nambiar and Seshadri, 2004).

The variations in the pattern of ageing and longevity of different individuals are due to the different types of stress and other factors they encounter during their adult life which affect the normal expression of genes required for adulthood to reduce/eliminate/avoid such stress would lead to healthy ageing and extend longevity (Kanungo, 2003).

Therapeutic lifestyle changes; especially advice of correct diet and physical activity is the call of the hour. Appropriate advice will not only help in controlling the biochemical indices of the 'moderate' or 'at risk' population, but will also bring down the worldwide burden of disease and disability in the aged population. This would inevitably reduce the government's expenditure on health and medicine.

References

Ahmed, F. (2002) "Novel Foods Across the Lifespan: From Infant Formula to Impact on Ageing". *Asia Pacific J Clin Nutr*, 11: S112–S116.

Blair, S.N. and S. Brodney. (1999) "Effects of Physical Inactivity and Obesity on Morbidity and Mortality: Current Evidence and Research Issues". *Med Sci Spiorts Exerc*, 31 (Suppl. 11): S646–S662.

Casperson, C.J., Bennie P.M. Bloemberg and H.M. Wim. (1991) "The Prevalence of Selected Physical Activities and their Relation with Coronary

Heart Disease Risk Factors in Elderly Men". *Am J Epidemiol*, 133: 1078–92.

Durnin, J.V.G.A. (1983) "Body Composition and Energy Expenditure in Elderly People". *Biblthca Nutr Dieta.*, 323: 16–30.

Forsen, T., J.G. Eriksson, J. Tuomilehto, C. Osmond and D.J. Barker. (1999) "Growth in Utero and during Childhood among Women Who Develop Coronary Heart Disease: Longitudinal Study". *BMJ*, 319: 1403–1407.

Gopalan, C. (1992) *Nutrition in Development Transition in South-East Asia*. WHO (SEARO), NFI Special Publication Series, New Delhi.

Gopalan, C. (1993) *Nutritive Value of Indian Foods*. National Institute of Nutrition, Hyderabad.

ICMR. (1989) Recommended Dietary Allowances for Indians, Indian Council of Medical Research, pp. 14–41.

Kanungo, M.N. (2003) "Biology of Ageing". *NFI Bulletin*, Vol. 24 (4): 7–8.

Langenberg, C., R. Hardy, D. Kuh, E. Brunner and M. Wadsworth. (2003) "Central and Total Obesity in Middle Aged Men and Women in Relation to Lifetime Socioeconomic Status: Evidence from a National Birth Cohort". *Journal of Epidemiology and Community Health*, 57: 816–822.

Mehta, Pallavi and V.S. Nambiar. (1999) *Ageing, Health and Nutrition*. Department of Foods and Nutrition, Faculty of Home Science, M.S. University of Baroda, Vadodara, pp. 1–51.

Misra, A. and L. Khurana. (2008) "Obesity and the Metabolic Syndrome in Developing Countries". *J Clin Endocrinol Metab*, 93 (Suppl. 11): S9–30.

Nambiar, V.S. and P. Guin. (2007) "Prevalence of Hyperglycemia and Hyperlipidemia Among the Middle Aged and Elderly Population in a University Setup". *Indian J Geron.*, 21 (1): 30–43.

Nambiar, V.S. and S. Seshadri. (2002) "Relationship between Socio-demographic Indicators, Income, Lifestyle and Caloric Intake in Postmenopausal Women". *Indian Journal of Gerontology*, Vol. 16, Nos. 3 and 4.

Nambiar, V.S. and S. Seshadri. (2004) "Dietary Patterns and its Relation to Disease Profile in Postmenopausal Women". (Part II), *Indian Journal of Gerontology*, Vol. 18 (8): 73–84.

Pan, X.R., G.W. Li, Y.H. Hu, J.X. Wang and Z.X. An. (1997) "Effect of Diet and Exercise in Preventing NIDDM in People with Impaired Glucose Tolerance: The Da Qing IGT and Diabetes Study". *Diabetes Care*, 20: 537–544.

Patel, V. and S. Seshadri. (1992) Nutritional Status of Women Aged 45–58 yr from Affluent and Middle Income Groups in an Urban Setting in India. Unpublished M.Sc (Nutrition) Dissertation, Department of Foods and Nutrition, M.S. University of Baroda, Vadodara.

Popkin, B.M. (1998) "The Nutrition Transition and its Health Implications in Lower-income Countries". *Public Health Nutr.*, 1: 5–21.

Popkin, B.M. (2001) "Nutrition Transition and Obesity in the Developing World". *Journal of Nutrition*, 131: 871S–873S.

Ramachandran, A., C. Snehalatha, A. Kapur, V. Vijaya, V. Mohan, A.K. Das et al. (2001). "High Prevalence of Diabetes and Impaired Glucose Tolerance in India: National Urban Diabetes Survey". *Diabetologia*, 44: 1094–1101.

Rosenberg, I.H. and J.W. Miller. (1992) "Nutritional Factors in Physical and Cognitive Function in the Elderly". *Am J Clin Nutr.*, 55: 1237S–1243S.

Solomons, N.W. (2002) "Nutrition and the Extremes of Life: Dilemmas and Enigmas of Advanced Age". *Asia Pacific J Clin Nutr.*, 11 (4): 247–250.

Solomons, N.W. and A.S. Anderson. (2002) "Diet, Lifestyle and Chronic Disease Risk: Assessing and Improving Strategies for Prevention Interventions, a Global Perspective". *Asia Pacific J Clin Nutr.*, 11: S779–S782.

Tucker, K.L. and S. Burnanapin. (2001) "Nutrition and Ageing in Developing Countries". *J Nutr*, 131: 2417S–2423S.

WHO Expert Consultation. (2004) Appropriate Body-Mass Index for Asian Populations and its Implications for Policy and Intervention Strategies". *Lancet*, 363 (9403): 157–63.

World Health Organization. (2005) A Report on Preventing Chronic Diseases: A Vital Investment.

http://www.nnmbindia.org/publications.html

11

Greying Community of India

VARSHA PARIKH

Ageing is a natural process that begins at birth, or to be more precise, at conception, a process that progresses throughout one's life and ends at death. It is a constant, predictable process that involves growth and development of living organisms. Ageing cannot be avoided, but how fast we age varies from one person to another. How we age depends upon our genes, environmental influences, and lifestyle. Ageing can be defined as a state of mind, which does not always keep pace with our chronological age. Attitude and how well we face the normal changes, challenges and opportunities of later life may best define our age.

As ageing is a continuous process in the structure and functions of the body, the physical abilities of the former tend to slow down with the passage of years. It is an impoverished environment, poor nutrition and diseases that breakdown the nervous system's natural potential resistance against deterioration. As far as the psychological structures and functions are concerned, these need not necessarily be deterioration. Thus, growing older cannot be prevented. One begins ageing at the time of conception and continues till death. However, some of the effects of ageing can be slowed and even prevented. Prevention in later years requires participating in health education and health promotion activities designed to reduce the risk of disease. Prevention also involves engaging in interventions that improve outcomes in the event an illness does occur and includes efforts that reduce the risk of progressive disability and decline of function. In later life the goals of prevention also include maintaining function, vitality and quality of life.

According to Wikipedia, ageing is any change in an organism over time. Ageing refers to a multidimensional process of physical, psychological, and social change (Hultsch and Deutsch). Some dimensions of ageing grow and expand over time, while others decline. Reaction time, for example, may slow with age, while knowledge of world events and wisdom may expand (Schaie). Research shows that even late in life potential exists for physical, mental, and social growth and development. Ageing is an important part of all human societies reflecting the biological changes that occur, but also reflecting cultural and societal conventions. Age is usually measured in full years—and months for young children. A person's birthday is often an important event.

Chronological ageing, referring to how old a person is, is arguably the most straightforward definition of ageing and may be distinguished from 'social ageing' (society's expectations of how people should act as they grow older) and 'biological ageing' (an organism's physical state as it ages). Stuart-Hamilton also notes distinction between 'proximal ageing' (age-based effects that come about because of factors in the recent past) and 'distal ageing' (age-based differences that can be traced back to a cause early in person's life, such as childhood poliomyelitis).

In all, human beings are inescapable to the process of ageing. Process of ageing slowly but surely decreases the individual's ability to cope with its environment. The ageing process can also be observed internally, i.e., in the changes of body composition, structural tissues and tissue cell loss and replacement.

Ageing and Demographic Transition

One of the major features of demographic transition in the world has been the considerable increase in the absolute and relative numbers of elderly people. Of the global population of over 6 billion almost 10 per cent are elderly. Further, it is projected that the older population in developing countries will rise much faster than the developed countries. This has been especially true in the case of developing countries like India also. About 60 per cent of the elderly live in the developing world, and this will rise to 70 per cent by 2010. Further, the older population itself is ageing, with the oldest old being more than 10 per cent of the world's elderly. In India, the proportion of older persons has risen from 4.9 per cent in 1901 to 5.5 per cent in 1951, 6.5 per cent in 1991, 7.7 per cent in 2001 and will be 12 per cent in 2025.

The demographic profile of aged in India 1991–2001 is presented in Table 1.

Table 1 *Demographic Profile of Aged in India 1991–2001*

States/Union Territories	2001		1991	
	Number in '000	Per cent to Total Population	Number in '000	Per cent to Total Population
A & N Islands	17	4.87	10	3.55
Andhra Pradesh	5,788	7.64	4,306	6.47
Arunachal Pradesh	50	4.57	37	4.33
Assam	1,560	5.86	1186	4.25
Bihar	5,501	6.64	5,227	6.05
Chandigarh	45	4.99	29	4.52
Chhatisgarh	1,504	7.23	NA	
Dadra and Nagar Haveli	9	4.00	6	4.40
Daman and Diu	8	5.09	6	6.32
Delhi	720	5.22	444	4.72
Goa	112	8.35	74	6.34
Gujarat	3,499	6.92	2,540	6.15
Haryana	1,584	7.51	1,230	7.42
Himachal Pradesh	548	9.01	402	7.79
Jammu & Kashmir	675	6.71	432	5.78
Jharkhand	1,579	5.87	NA	
Karnataka	4,062	7.70	3,041	6.78
Kerala	3,336	10.48	2,549	8.77
Lakshadweep	4	6.15	3	5.22
Madhya Pradesh	4,281	7.09	4,254	6.43
Maharashtra	8,455	8.74	5,453	6.91
Manipur	145	6.09	109	5.94
Meghalaya	106	4.58	82	4.62
Mizoram	49	5.50	34	4.93

Cont'd...

Cont'd...

Nagaland	90	4.54	65	5.40
Orissa	3,039	8.28	2,217	6.98
Pondicherry	81	8.32	56	6.90
Punjab	2,192	9.02	1,532	7.56
Rajasthan	3,810	6.75	2,666	6.06
Sikkim	29	5.37	19	4.66
Tamil Nadu	5,507	8.87	4,073	7.29
Tripura	233	7.29	192	6.96
Uttar Pradesh	11,649	7.02	9,250	6.65
Uttaranchal	584	6.89	NA	
West Bengal	5,700	7.11	4,087	6

Source: Prasad, Syam, http://mpra.ub.uni-muenchen.de/5935/2/MPRA_paper_5935.pdf.).

The process of ageing of population in India have regional dimensions and remains at differential stages of demographic transition. Among the states, Uttar Pradesh led with 11 million the elderly, followed by Maharashtra (8.5 million), Andhra Pradesh and West Bengal (5.7 million each) and Bihar and Tamil Nadu with 5.5 million each. The smallest number of the elderly is found in the union territory of Lakshadweep. The low fertility state of Kerala ranks as number one with the highest proportion of the elderly in the country with 10.5 in 2001. Punjab and Himachal Pradesh occupy the second largest position in terms of per cent of the elderly, followed by states of Tamil Nadu (8.9) and Maharashtra (8.7). Dadra and Nagar Haveli registered the lowest proportion (4). The highest per cent of 80 years and above is seen in Himachal Pradesh (1.3%), followed by Kerala (1.2%).

With a fast increasing trend, India's the elderly population aged 60 and above is expected to increase from 77 million in 2001 to 179 million in 2031 and further to 301 million in 2051. The proportion is likely to reach 12 per cent in 2031 and 17 per cent in 2051. The number of the elderly persons above 70 years of age (old-old) is likely to increase more sharply than of the elderly above 60 years and above. The old-old are projected to increase fivefold between 2001–2051 (from 29 million in 2001 to 132 million in 2051). Their proportion is expected to rise from 2.9 to 7.6 per cent. Although we have found excess males in the age group 60 and above, the old-old sex ratio is very favourable to females. The oldest old (80+) among the elderly in India is expected to grow faster than any other age group in the population. In absolute terms, it is likely to increase fourfold from 8 million in 2001 to 32 million in 2051. In short, India is dooming towards a greying future (Rajan, 2006). This indeed indicate need to pay attention for this group of the Indian society.

This change in the age distribution contributing to longevity can be attributed to following main factors:

- Available and effective health care (medical training in disabilities, better nutrition, disease prevention).
- Research about growing older (richer medical and social science literature enabling better services).
- Cohort differences (40-year-olds born in the 1960s—different life experiences).
- Public policy attention (governmental financing of services, laws, regulations).
- Education (academic interest in gerontology and greater awareness among administrators, educators, and professionals) as suggested by demographers and researchers.
- The older population will increase dramatically in the next 10–20 years.
- Current and future older adults will be healthier and better educated than previous generations, and
- There is a low expectation that families will be able to absorb all the older persons who will need care at home.

Elderly Status in the Indian Society

There are 8 million older people in India – 11 lakh in Delhi itself. According to an estimate nearly 40 per cent of senior citizens living with their families are reportedly facing abuse of one kind or another, but only one in six cases actually comes to light. Although the President has given her assent to the Maintenance and Welfare of Parents and Senior Citizens Act (2006) which punishes children who abandon parents with a prison term of three months or a fine, situation is grim for elderly people in India.

The inescapable fact remains that wherever there is functional decline and debility, the quality of life does get compromised. Economic dependence and social restriction further adds to the gravity of situation. Being cut off from the professional, occupational, social-neighbourhood, environ and even from the busy near and dear ones may serve as the last straw on the breaking back. The dilemma of dichotomy of longevity on one hand and an enormously compromised quality of life on the other is indeed perplexing.

The National Sample Survey Organization (NSSO), which is a division of the Department of Statistics operating within the Ministry of Planning and Programme Implementation, is a nodal statistical agency of the Government of India. The NSSO, conducted a survey on aged persons between July, 1995 and June, 1996. In the survey, data on the number of living children of the aged, their living arrangement, state of economic independence, number of dependants, person supporting the aged, disability, chronic ailments, state of health and their familial roles in the household were collected. Information was also gathered on the routine activities of the elderly, retirement benefits, provisions for regular income, etc. The samples were chosen through a stratified two-stage design. Finally, 12,614 village/urban blocks with 1,20,942 households and 33,981 aged were surveyed from the whole country. Some major findings of the status of the elderly in India are as follows:

- There are more elderly in rural areas. There is also movement of the elderly from urban to rural areas.
- Old age dependency is higher in rural areas than in urban areas.
- The elderly are ageing.
- There are more females than males among the aged and in contrast to the general sex ratios are rising.
- The elderly are much less literate and educated than the general population.
- The elderly generally live with their spouses/children and other relatives, however more and more elderly are now living without their children.
- As many as 70 per cent of the aged depend on others for their day-to-day maintenance. The situation is far worse for elderly females, 85 to 87 per cent of whom are dependent on others.
- A majority of the elderly are not supported by any retirement benefits and the problem is compounded in rural areas.
- About 54 per cent of the aged own financial assets and housing, though many of them do not have any management rights or control over them.

- The prevalence of chronic diseases among the aged is quite high and it is higher still in urban areas. Problems of the joints and throat are the most common.
- The prevalence of disability among the aged is also very high.
- A great majority of the elderly participate in social and religious matters and in household chores, though a large number of them cannot participate in household activities.

With reference to Elderly Status Index (ESI), covering factors viz., life expectancy at age 60, literacy, living arrangements, economic independence, retirement benefits, ownership and control of wealth, health status and social interaction indicates that, there is no data on healthy life expectancy for Indian states. The ESI has been estimated from above NSS data which indicates that the elderly are most well placed in Himachal Pradesh followed by Punjab and Jammu & Kashmir. The elderly status is lowest in Assam, preceded by Karnataka. The index shows that in the urban areas, the elderly in Kerala enjoy a slightly better status than their counterparts in West Bengal (Chakraborty, 2004).

Problems of Greying Community in India

Ageing is an universal phenomenon, however, it is noted fact that becoming old invites various kinds of problems. Ageing has a charming beginning in the form of development, it has a dismal end marked by senescency, loss of adaptability of the organism to its extrinsic and intrinsic environments, decrepitude and ultimately the mecabre death. Thus, the problems of olds are differ than the problems of youths.

Various authors, viz., Sahu (1998), Joshi (1971), Cheriboga (1982) and many others have reported about the problems of greying community in India. These studies lead to conclude that with ageing there is decline in many functions which led to feelings of inadequacy and insecurity. Social isolation in old age is also caused by several factors. All these shows that, various issues related to social, physical, economical dimension of aged life gradually starts cropping up. Above studies also shows that the greying community of India suffers from various kinds of problems such as physical health problems, economic problems, social problem and miscellaneous problem.

Physical Health Problems

Physical health problems increase with age. Elderly people are more likely to have major health concerns than the rest of the population.

Hence, problem of health is very important to the aged people. During the old age, power of resisting a diseases diminishes. They became ill due to the frequent attack of various diseases and no medicine can cure them completely. The old people become home-bound due to their dim eyesight, hearing deficiency and poor physique. Thus, after a certain age health problems begin to crop up leading to losing control over one's body, even not recognizing own family owing to Alzheimer are common in old age. It is then children began to see their parents as burden. It is these parents who at times wander out of their homes or are thrown out. Some dump their old parents or grandparents in old-age homes and do not even come to visit them anymore. For instance, Delhi has nearly 11 lakh senior citizens but there are only four governments-run homes for them and 31 by NGOs, private agencies and charitable trusts. The facilities are lacking in government-run homes.

The WHO reports physical health concerns in the following areas increases due to the ageing:

- Physical deconditioning and loss of stamina
- Obesity-related diseases
- Sensory impairments
- Poly-pharmacy and adverse medication reactions
- Mobility impediments
- Tobacco or second-hand smoke
- Exposure to toxicity in work place
- Contagious diseases
- Abuse and violence
- Poor nutrition (lack of availability or by choice)
- Non-medical drug use
- Passive lifestyle

R.D. Chakraborty (2004) reported about the NSS data of 1995–96 in his book. The National Sample Survey (1995–96) provides a clear picture of chronic diseases from which aged people in India suffered the most. The prevalence of chronic diseases among the aged was in general seen to be very high. Chronic diseases in complicated health areas were higher in the urban areas. This was found in an Economic and Social Commission for Asia and the Pacific (ESCAP) study too. Further in India, problems of the joints and throat happened to be the most severe diseases for the aged. Blood pressure problem came next. Lifestyle diseases like heart diseases, urinary infections and diabetes appeared to have taken considerable place in the suffering pattern of the people. Further, ageing also bring with it various forms of physical disability, viz., visual disability, hearing disability, speech disability and locomotor disability generally found the most. The findings from the National Sample Survey reveal that around 40 per cent of the rural aged and 35 per cent of the urban aged suffer physical disabilities. Visual disability was mentioned by about 24–27 per cent of the aged and half of these people also suffered hearing disabilities. The females suffered from more disabilities than the males. Visual disability had the highest incidence, failing eyesight is concomitant with ageing. The NFHS data shows that blindness is highest among the elderly. Further, study reflect that 12 to 15 per cent of older people are said to have a hearing impairment in both urban and rural areas. Locomotor disabilities usually are a result of paralysis, dysfunction of limbs, amputation or dystrophy of joints. The disabled elderly require more intense support than the elderly suffering from a chronic illness.

Economical Problems

The National Sample Survey collected data on the economic dependence of the elderly in India, shows that as many as 70 per cent of the aged had to depend on others for their livelihood. The situation was worse for elderly females. Over 85 per cent were found to be dependent, partially or fully on others. The situation was slightly better in the urban areas than the national average, but the rural elderly virtually are at the mercy of others. R.D. Chakraborty (2004) stated that the determinant of changing social relationships are very complex but demographics are certainly influential. As fewer children support parents for longer periods of time, the per capita cost of 'parent caring' is high. The tremendous jump in health care costs, unaccompanied by suitable development of health insurance schemes, multiples the burden of children. All these lead children to choose not to fulfil the implicit obligation to care for their elderly parents.

Social Problems

Chakraborty (2004) states that participation in social, household and religious activities is essential for the well-being of all ages. Connecting with family members, friends, neighbours, work colleagues and community groups brings happiness to all. In older ages this is more important, since older people are more likely to lose loved ones and friends, and are therefore more vulnerable to loneliness, social isolation and availability of a 'smaller social pool'. Social isolation in old age is linked to a decline in both physical and mental capacities and an increase in health damaging behaviours such as excessive alcohol consumption and physical inactivity.

Graceful Ageing

However, ageing is not a crisis: society and the economy will be able to adjust to changing circumstances. Healthy ageing is becoming an increasingly important issue for older persons, the public focus on maintaining the aged has sometimes fostered a negative image of ageing. Older people have spent a long life on this earth. A reinterpretation of their life stories provides us with an opportunity to examine our lives in retrospect, to correct some of our past actions. However, to ensure a healthy, independent, quality life in older age, graceful ageing by optimizing opportunities for physical, social and mental well-being throughout life is not difficult to offer to those need. Thus, factors that can enhance quality of life could be requiring to have joint venture of aged person, their family as well as the society as a whole. Above issues require strategic efforts to address it. It can be effectively deal as follows:

- Social planning
- Planning for ageing population
- Identifying who are the older adults and careers
- Determining what they may need
- Looking at demographic trends recognizing that needs are often linked to age (younger-older vs older-older)
- Thinking in terms of creative approaches to support
- Involving the families in the planning
- Working with government for institution of universal models for helping families and people with disabilities
- Factors affecting planning
- Dynamics of population demographics—how they change?
- Economic security—extant pensions and financial aid to people with disabilities
- Presence or lack of 'ageing-friendly' communities and neighbourhoods
- Public policy focus with increasing age-aging or disability?
- Governmental policies and commitment to solving long-term or future problems—what level and whether legislative or administrative?

Some of the ways through which the aged can enhance their quality of life are as follows:

Self-support by the Aged

It is a wrong notion that old people cannot adjust to lifestyle changes. Following are some of the do's that can help an aged to come across his path successfully:

- Exercise and fitness
- Healthy eating/reducing smoking and alcohol
- Stable affiliation with physician, clinic, or other health care centre
- Periodic health screening for ageing related conditions or diseases
- Early medical attention and special care for physical, dental, mental disability
- Social involvement
- Network of friends and involvement in life of community
- Accessible and affordable housing
- Help with shopping and other daily activities/Work or other challenging activities
- Recreational outlets (active and passive)
- Valued status by community
- Partnerships, planning, and improving quality of life
- Aid with finding employment
- Self-advocacy for meeting needs

Family and Societal Support

A probable solution to the lifelong factors help produce an healthier old age is the multidimensional approach that comprises not only curative but also non-curative methods of care that are essentially preventive, rehabilitative and ones that pertain to terminal and respite care.

The elderly, being less able to be independent, need the care and support of others in several respects. Taking care of the elderly refers mainly to the emotional support; on the other hand, support given to the elderly refers to the financial and material support. The former type of support is expected from the families or persons closer; whereas the latter is supposed to be a joint effort of the immediate family and society. The care and support enjoyed by the elderly is linked to their residence. Here family is the safest form of security and rates living alone removed from there immediate relatives (spouse and child) as the biggest form of deprivation for the elderly. Further, Indian elderly live in extended multigenerational households and rely primarily on their adult children for financial support and personal care. It is the family members and neighbours who provide the bulk of the support and care to older adults who need assistance. However, these traditional families are now showing signs of breaking up due to demographic, economic and social change, there is no replacement for the family as a source of support for the elderly. The aged do not have the resources or the ability to support themselves. Thus, family has to act as an important partner for offering graceful ageing to Indian elders. In this reference, these families also can be supported, motivated and encouraged by the state if they are to continue to provide care and support to the elderly without becoming over-burdened in the process.

Government Support for Elderly

Graceful ageing requires elderly-friendly and supportive economic, physical and social environments. Some of the national level policies offered to elderly in India are as follows:

- Legal arrangements made by the Indian states to protect the elderly—The Himachal Pradesh government and Government of Maharashtra passed a parents maintenance bill wherein a simple procedure was introduced for parents being ignored by their children to be given maintenance.
- National policy on older persons—The Government of India announced a National Policy on Older Persons (NPOP) in January 1999 which identified a number of areas of intervention-financial security, health care and nutrition, shelter, education, welfare, protection of life and property for the well-being of older persons in the country.
- A National Council for Older Persons (NCOP) was constituted by the Ministry of Social Justice and Empowerment to operationalize the National Policy on Older Persons. Rights of the elderly are clearly depicted as listed below:

— Parents cannot be evicted from a house without due process of law if they have been staying therefrom before. There are three enactments that can be applied:

(i) Under section 125 of the CRPC, a magistrate can order a child to maintain his old parents under the Maintenance of Parents Act.

(ii) The Hindu Adoptions and Maintenance Act says an aged parent can demand maintenance from children in the same way that a wife can demand it from her husband.

(iii) The Domestic Violence Act too provides parents with the right to seek relief from any kind of abuse.

Some of the national level programmes offered to elderly in India are as follows:

- Old Age Social and Income Security (OASIS): The growing concern for old age social and income security due to changes in demographic, social and traditional structures, the Social Defence Bureau had commissioned the national project titled Old Age Social and Income Security (OASIS)
- Integrated Programme for Older Persons: An integrated programme for older persons has been formulated by revising the earlier scheme of assistance to voluntary organizations for programmes relating to the welfare of the aged.
- Scheme of assistance for construction of old age homes: The scheme aims at providing a grant for the construction of old age home or service centres for older persons.
- National Old Age Pension Scheme: This scheme is implemented in the state and union territories through panchayats and municipalities.
- Old age and widow pension in different states of India: The states like Maharashtra, Karnataka, West Bengal, Kerala provides pension to the widows. However, each of the state has its own criteria.

Conclusion

The aim of development is to improve the well-being of the entire population on the basis of its full participation in the process of development and an equitable distribution of the benefits that are generated in the process. The development process must enhance human dignity and ensure equity among all age groups in the sharing of society's resources, rights and responsibilities. An important objective of socio-economic development is an age-integrated society, in which age discrimination and involuntary segregation is eliminated and in which solidarity and mutual support among generations is encouraged. Ageing is a lifelong process and should be recognized as such. The preparation of the entire population for later stages of life should be an integral part of social policies and encompass physical, psychological, cultural, religious, economic, health and other factors. Ageing in addition to being a symbol of experience and wisdom, can bring human beings closer to personal fulfilment, according to their beliefs and aspirations.

Bibliography

Chakraborty, R.D. (2004) *Population Ageing in the Context of Asia*. Sage Publications, New Delhi.

Irudaya Rajan, S., U.S. Mishra and P.S. Sarma. (1999) *India's Elderly: Burden or Challenge?* Sage Publications, New Delhi.

Kasthoori, R. (1996) *The Problems of the Aged: A Sociological Study*. Uppal Publishing House, New Delhi.

Kohli, A.S. (1996) *Social Situation of the Aged in India*. Anmol Publications Pvt. Ltd., New Delhi.

Mishra, S. (1987) *Social Adjustment in Old Age*. B.R. Publishing Corporation, Delhi.

Sahu, C. (1998) *Problems of Ageing among the Indian Tribes*. Sarup and Sons, New Delhi.

Webliography

http://74.125.153.132/search?q=cache:VLo_EtL5HAJ:www.hkcss.org.hk/rh/1_Professor_Janicki_Hong_Kong-aging-general-6%2729%2709.ppt+ageing+ needs+and+issues&cd=28&hl=en&ct= clnk&gl=in&client=firefox

http://www.azadindia.org/social-issues/problem-of-old-age-in-india.html

http://74.125.153.132/search?q=cache:5_IReGdrGc0J:www.japi.org/october2005/E843.pdf+issues+of+elderly+in+India&cd=1&hl=en&ct=clnk&gl=in&client=firefox

http://74.125.153.132/search?q=cache:RwqJpE0Ca8gJ:mpra.ub.uni-muenchen.de/5935/2/MPRA_paper_5935.pdf+active+elderly+in+India&cd=15&hl=en&ct=clnk&gl=in&client=firefox

12

Role and Status of Aged Women

An Analysis of Preferred and Performed Home Role

MINAXI PATHAK, IRA BORA AND RUPLEKHA BORAH

Human beings proceed through a predictable course of biological development leading from infancy to children on to adolescence and youth, then to adulthood and middle age and finally to old age and ultimate extinction. The term aged, elderly on senior citizens is used to describe a section of human population, usually refers to a particular group of person who have reached a certain chronological age. Age definition and differentiation carry significance to the society and the individual.

Traditionally, in India, the aged enjoyed place of honour and respect in the family and community and were treated as repositories of experience, skill and wisdom. With the breaking up of joint family system, the knowledge and experience of the old people loss significance in the proper functioning of society. The younger generation replaces the aged people in their powerful positions, leaving them in a weekend and functionless situation. In consequences, there is a decline in role and status of aged population in the present society. Today, a sizeable proportion of them are viewed as non-productive and have become highly dependent. In India low income and poverty-ridden life make elder persons dependent on their family members. It has been observed that older sector of population is the fastest growing segment of the world's population and it is in the developing region where the increase is the most rapid. The advancement of physical and medical sciences, economic development, rapid expansion of public health services along with social welfare and social security measures have resulted in increase of life expectancy. It has brought about a demographic transition leading to sharp increase in the population of the aged. Family is considered to be the most important social unit that has special significance for aged people. Activities performed by aged women and their status may vary with socio-economic status, employment status, locality, geographic conditions, etc. Kaur and Kaur (1987) observed that majority of aged women had say in important family matters such as children's education, children's marriage, household expenditure, religious work and dealing with relatives. Parthasarathy (1980) reported that some research workers had detected a declining status in old people in present family compositions. Again, due to factor of ageing, they appeared to command less importance by younger generation in the family and also other family members.

With the development of social services and a greater thrust on human resource development, the children, youth and women become the participants and targets of the development process. The aged continue to be neglected and are the recipients of only welfare services. The aged should not be viewed as a problem, but also as a precious resources, which should be harnessed for promoting the economic and social development of the community. Considering the importance of the elderly in the Indian society and their past contributions, the study is undertaken with an aim to throw light upon status and role of aged women, so that their potentialities could be utilized in full form. Various developmental programmes may be planned with the aged women in which their preference may be honoured with a view to make these resource more productive.

Objectives of the Study

- To study the status of aged women as reflected in family decision-making.
- To explore home role preferred and home role performed by the aged women in respect to selected activities.

Materials and Methods

A multi-stage sampling procedure was followed in the present study. The sampling design was purposive-cum-random sampling for descriptive survey. In the first stage, six municipality wards were selected randomly in Nowgong district of Assam. Households having joint family system were selected purposively from six wards and 100 respondents at the age group of 60 and above were selected following purposive-cum-random sampling method.

Interview method was the data gathering instrument for the present study. The schedule was developed keeping in view the objectives of the study. The interview schedule complied of three parts. Part I contained questions on personal and demographic characteristics of the aged females, part II contained statement about status of aged women as reflected by family decision-making regarding food, clothing, housing, education, financial matters and social activities while part III included statements about role preferred and performed by the aged women in the selected areas.

Analysis of data comprised of coding, categorization, tabulation and statistical analysis. To determine the status of the of the aged women in family decision-making, the items of decision-making areas were scored on the basis of frequency of consultation, i.e., always, sometimes and never through 2, 1 and 0 respectively. Data were analysed by calculating mean, standard deviation and standard error and status of the aged women were categorized as high, medium and low. '*t*' test was computed to test the significant relationship between the variables.

Results and Discussion

Personal and Demographic Characteristics

Data pertaining to personal and demographic characteristics of aged women revealed that more than 50 per cent respondents belonged to 60–65 years and about one fourth respondents were 71 years and above. Majority of the respondents (64%) were widow. Education level of the aged females indicated that primary school and middle school education were common, however one-fifth of the females were illiterate. This may be due to the fact that prior to independence, women education was neglected. The present occupational status of the aged women revealed that 87 per cent were housewives and 13 per cent were teachers in primary schools.

As far as personal income of the respondents was concerned, it was observed that 61 per cent had no income and were dependent on sons, while 39 per cent had some sources of income ranging from less than Rs 1,000 to 5,000 and above. Analysis of various sources of income showed that pension (own and husband) were the prime source for 29 per cent of the aged women followed by farm/business income (10%), self-employment (7%) and rental property (4%).

Demographic characteristics pertaining to the religion, caste, type and size of the family, occupation and family income of the respondents families were studied. A large majority of the respondents (90%) were Hindus and 56 per cent belonged to general castes. Nearly three-fourth of the respondents were from extended families with seven to ten members. Data on family income revealed that about three-fourth of the respondents households (72%) belonged to middle income group (Rs 10,001 to Rs 15,000) and 17 per cent belonged to low income group (below Rs 10,000), while 11 per cent were from high income group (above Rs 15,001).

Status of Aged Females in Family Decision-making

Status of aged women in the family was studied in terms of their frequency of consultation in family decision-making which includes food and non-food items, academic matter of grandchildren, financial matters and social activities of the family. Fifty per cent respondents desired to get involved in family decision-making as they were interested to play an active role in family decisions while 36 per cent felt that involvement in family decision-making could make them well informed, 5 per cent respondents were interested to share their experiences with the family members while making decisions and only 9 per cent felt that there was no need to counsel them.

Decision-making Regarding Food, Clothing and Housing

Food, clothing and housing are the basic necessities of human life. So these are the important decision-making areas in families. Among these three areas, housing was the major area where a majority of the aged females were invariably consulted by the family members (65%) followed by food (61%). In clothing, consultation with the aged females was relatively less (14%). Further analyses of data showed that in the area of food, aged females were consulted in selection of menu (70%) followed by method of preparation (68%). In the area of clothing decisions, three-fourth of the respondents

were sometimes consulted in clothing purchase for specific occasions. It was observed that aged female played a vital role in dressing decision. They were mostly consulted in case of renovation (74%), repairing (74%) purchasing of land (62%), selling of land (54%) and painting/white washing (70%). This may be because of the fact that most of the aged females were the owners of the house or land.

Decision-making Regarding Education Family Members

Data as regards to decision of education of grandchildren revealed that majority of the aged women were never (70.8%) consulted as far as academic matters of grandchildren was concerned. The areas in which majority of aged women were 'never' consulted were age of sending grandchildren to school (65%), selection of medium of education (67%), selection of school (65%), selection of extra-curricular activities (88%) and selection of career of grandchildren (69%). It may be due to the fact that most of the respondents were less educated.

Decision-making Regarding Financial Matters

In case of economic decisions, majority of aged women were 'never' consulted (76.80%). It may be because of the reason that most of the respondents were financially dependent, hence decisions regarding savings, credits paying loan, etc., were solely taken by their sons or daughter-in-laws without consulting their mothers. This findings is in agreement with the findings of Ahuja et al. (2000) in which only 6.67 per cent of the aged women played dominant role in financial decisions in Punjab.

Decision-making Regarding Social Activities

Social activities were major family activities in sample households. It was encouraging to note that majority of the aged females were always consulted (82.6%). Itemwise analysis showed that aged women were 'always' consulted in case of marriage of grandchildren (100%), celebration of festivals (91%), attending social ceremonies (79%) and for entertaining guests (77%). On the whole, aged women played an important role in decision-making as regards to social activities, housing and food related matters. However they had little role to play in financial matters and education of grandchildren.

On the basis of the scores on frequency of consultation with the aged women in the areas of food, clothing, housing, education, financial and social decisions, status of the aged females was categorized as high, medium and low. It was encouraging to note that maximum percentages of respondents were categorized as having high status (42%), 21 per cent were in medium status and 37 per cent aged women had low status in decision-making (Table 1). Hence, it was observed that Assamese aged females had played considerably an important role in family decision-making.

Table 1 *Distribution of Aged Women as per their Status in Decision-making*

Scores	*Characteristics*	*Percentage*
>57.35	High status	42
Between 57.35 and 53.27	Medium status	21
<53.27	Low status	37

Mean = 28.22, S.D.= 10.35, S.E. 1.04.

Home Role Preferred and Performed by the Aged Women

In the present study, home role means work performed by the women in relation to their position in the household in the areas of food preparation, child and family care, housekeeping and social and leisure time activities with a view to manage the home effectively.

Food Preparation Activities

Data pertaining to role preferred and role performed by aged women revealed that majority of the respondents preferred food related activities. Itemwise analysis shows that preparation activities, cooking and serving food were the must preferred activities as expressed by 73 per cent, 64 per cent, 68 per cent of the respondents respectively. As far as performance was concerned, mostly performed activities were pre-preparation activities (44%), cooking food (43%) and serving food (43%). Fetching water and grinding flours and masalas were 'never' preferred and performed by the most of the aged women (50% and 57%, respectively) (Table 2).

Table 2 *Food Preparation Activities Preferred and Performed by Aged Women*

(N=100)

Food Preparation Activities	*Preferred*				*Performed*			
	M	*S*	*R*	*N*	*M*	*S*	*R*	*N*
Pre-preparation activities	73	18	3	6	44	25	15	16
Cooking	69	20	3	8	43	19	13	25
Serving food	68	19	3	10	43	17	13	27
Grinding masalas	34	9	8	49	16	13	14	57
Fetching water from well	23	9	5	63	9	16	7	68
Preparation of milk products—boiling milk	51	28	5	16	34	33	9	24
Preparation of jam/jelly	47	22	4	27	32	27	4	37
Mean	52.14	17.86	4.43	25.57	31.57	21.43	10.71	36.29

M= Mostly, S= Sometimes, R= Rarely, N= Never.

Child and Family Care Activities

A large majority of the aged females mostly preferred looking after family members (92%), taking care of sick grandchildren (93%). Accordingly more than 70 per cent got involved in these activities which implies that aged females got scope for performing the activities as per her preference (Table 3). The activities like preparation of supplementary foods for grandchildren, feeding, massaging/bathing/dressing grandchildren, more than 65 per cent women often preferred to perform, wherein in case of performance, they did not get the scope to be involved frequently. This may be due to the reason that daughter-in-laws enjoyed these activities and preferred to handle the children's personal activities themselves. Paying attention to homeworks of grandchildren, accompanying grandchildren to school and immunization of grandchildren were neither preferred nor performed mostly by the aged women. As majority of the aged women were less educated, they might lack confidence in preferring activities related to child's education and health.

Table 3 *Child and Family Care Activities Preferred and Performed by Aged Women*

(N=100)

Child and Family Care Activities	Preferred				Performed			
	M	S	R	N	M	S	R	N
Preparation of food for children	56	24	10	10	40	32	6	22
Feeding grandchildren	65	22	—	13	35	34	8	23
Bathing grandchildren	45	23	10	22	34	35	8	23
Teaching children good practices/telling stories	78	15	2	5	68	21	3	8
Paying attention to homework	15	8	3	74	4	9	13	74
Accompanying grandchildren to school	3	13	14	70	1	6	13	80
Immunizing grandchildren	18	13	4	65	6	14	19	69
Taking care of sick grandchildren	93	5	—	2	74	10	10	6
Taking care of family members	92	5	—	3	71	13	10	6
Mean	61.82	11.64	1.18	25.36	46	18.45	5.50	30.5

M= Mostly, S= Sometimes, R= Rarely, N= Never.

Housekeeping Activities

Data related to role performed and role preferred by the aged women regarding housekeeping activities were presented in Table 4. It was observed that very few of the housekeeping activities were preferred as performed by the aged women. Most preferred activities were making beds for self (74%), supervision of household task performed by servants (56%). The least preferred activities were care of clothes, care of utensils, accountkeeping and shopping. More than 60 per cent aged women had never performed these activities. Activities related to household cleaning were somewhat preferred by the respondents, however majority of the respondents 'never' performed these activities (69%). It is because of the fact that these activities did not match with the age and status of the aged women. Further, work culture of the society also act as governing factor in determining the type of work to be performed.

Table 4 *Housekeeping Activities Preferred and Performed by Aged Women*

(N=100)

Housekeeping Activities	*Preferred*				*Performed*			
	M	*S*	*R*	*N*	*M*	*S*	*R*	*N*
Care of house	20	23	14	43	5	23	11	61
Care of clothes	16	14	25	45	6	16	9	69
Care of utensils	17	24	15	44	6	22	12	59
Making beds for self	74	16	2	8	29	47	4	20
Supervision of household task	56	40	—	4	48	10	38	4
Supervision of household repairs	18	14	3	65	14	13	3	32
Shopping for family members	18	14	3	65	14	13	3	66
Storing grocery	27	35	3	35	17	14	3	66
Accountkeeping	29	5	1	65	27	4	2	67
Saving for future	38	1	—	61	37	1	—	62
Average	25	15.68	6	51.42	15.37	15.63	6.53	60.58

M= Mostly, S= Sometimes, R= Rarely, N= Never.

Leisure Time Activities

Data as regards to preference of leisure time activities by aged women revealed that large majority of women had preference for social and religions activities like performing Puja (100%), celebrating festivals (95%), entertaining guests (93%), attending ceremonies (90%), visiting relatives and neighbours (89%). Accordingly, in the case of performance of these activities, a large majority of respondents mostly got involved in these activities either regularly or occasionally. Aged women preferred to perform the recreational activities like watching TV, reading books, magazines, newspapers, gardening, listening to holy songs. As far as performance was concerned, majority of them performed activities as their preference. Least preferred and performed leisure time activities were knitting, handloom weaving and embroidery (67%). Poor eyesight was the reason given by most of the aged women for not preferring these activities (Table 5).

Table 5 *Leisure Time Activities Preferred and Performed by Aged Women*

(N=100)

Leisure Time Activities	*Preferred*				*Performed*			
	M	*S*	*R*	*N*	*M*	*S*	*R*	*N*
Performing puja	100	—	—	—	1.00	—	—	—
Celebrating festivals	95	2	2	1	75	17	5	3
Entertaining guests	93	6	1	—	74	17	9	—
Attending ceremonies	90	3	1	6	53	31	11	5
Visiting friends and neighbours	89	4	2	5	57	27	10	6
Reading books/newspaper	72	7	2	19	61	9	6	24
Watching TV/dramas	81	8	5	6	76	13	5	6
Listening to devoted song/music	60	19	3	18	55	26	3	16
Knitting/weaving/ embroidery	15	30	1	54	19	11	3	67
Kitchen gardening	47	26	2	25	33	26	5	36
Supervision of works	60	18	1	21	43	16	5	36
Mean	71.0	11.69	2	15.31	56.23	16.77	6.62	20.38

M= Mostly, S= Sometimes, R=Rarely, N=Never.

Further analysis showed that there was a significant difference between role preference and their role performance of aged women as regards to food preparation activities (t value = 8.07** significant at 0.01 level), child and family care activities (t value = 11.2** significant at 0.01 level), housekeeping activities (t value = 4.44** significant at 0.01 level) and leisure time activities (t value 5.15** significant at 0.01 level). This indicates that although aged women occupied a high status in decision-making, performance of household activities were not according to their preference. The reasons may be attributed to health, generation gap and active involvement of other family member in performance of these activities.

Conclusions

Overall picture indicated that leisure time activities were mostly preferred and performed by the aged women followed by food preparation activities, child and family care activities. Housekeeping activities were least preferred and performed activities by the aged women. Efforts should be made by the family members to provide opportunities to the elderly for fruitful engagement. Also, elderly women with specialized skills, experiences and their preferences need to be identified to engage them according to their capabilities in various social welfare programmes. Social scientists, academicians, non-government organizations with their concerted efforts may create a conducive environment where elderly citizens could be engaged both for the benefit of the individual and community as a whole.

References

Ahuja, M., M.S. Dhillon and M.S. Sandhu. (2000) "An Analysis on the Life Satisfaction of Elderly in Rural Punjab". *Indian Psychological Review*, 54 (1 and 2): 27–33.

Dey, S. and K. Oberoi. (1990) "Psychological Problems of Old People in Rural and Urban Communities". *Maharashtra Journal of Extension Education*, IX: 331–333.

Kaur, S. and M. Kaur. (1987) "Psychological Problems of the Aged", in M.L. Sharma and T.M. Dak (eds.), *Ageing in India: Challenges for the Society*. Ajanta Publications, New Delhi, XVIII, 76–81.

Mishra, S. (1987) *Social Adjustment in Old Age*. B.R. Publishing Corporation, New Delhi.

Parthasarthy, N.R. (1980) "On Some Aspects of Ageing in India". *The Journal of Social Work*, XL (4): 381–386.

Swaminathan, D. (1996) "Integration of the Aged into Development Process in India". *Research and Development Journal*, 2 (2): 3–6.

13

Mismatch between Anthropometric Measurements and Dimensions of Toilet Chair

A Cause of Accidents

NIRMAL KAUR AND PROMILA SHARMA

It has been seen that the total number of accidents in the home takes place with the highest occurrences in the toilets, bathroom, kitchens and stairs.

Changes in body composition are well known to occur with old age, but there is limited knowledge of the rate of changes in anthropometric indices of body composition or the distribution of these changes in the elderly. The anthropometric standards derived from adult population may not be appropriate for the elderly because of body changes occurring during ageing. Specific anthropometric reference data for the elderly are necessary, before designing any kind of product or furniture or similar related equipment.

Bone, muscle and other minute and detailed dimensions of anatomy are mostly referred for medical and other necessities. But even while designing products for human use, the body dimension is of importance and the anthropometry has to be considered. The study of anthropometry is not just about body measurements, it is about how to employ body measurement information efficiently. While designing individual items or products one has to take into consideration the dimensions of the product, their layout pattern in a given space, than use, etc., to match with anthropometry of the user. Anthropometry includes measurements of body parts, strength, etc.

Hence, in the present study, some important and necessary anthropometric measurements were taken.

Objectives

1. To collect the anthropometric data of the people of third age.
2. To compare locally available toilet chair and ergonomically designed toilet chair.

Methodology

In the present study experimental design was planned to study anthropometric measurements for checking the difference between both kinds of toilet chair.

Selection of Locale and Sample

The present study was conducted in two regions of Uttarakhand state, i.e., Pantnagar and Rudrapur block of Udham Singh Nagar district. The whole list of families of Pantnagar and Rudrapur block was used to sort out the third age people, than out of that list the families were chosen randomly until the total sample size of 100 people each from both the blocks were selected. Now there were 100 third age people from each blocks, out of which 50 per cent were male and 50 per cent were female selected thus altogether making total sample size of 200 people of third age.

Measures

Anthropometric measurements like (sitting height, sitting shoulder height, popliteal height, buttock popliteal length, hip breadth and elbow rest height) and toilet chair dimensions like (extended backrest height, backrest height, seat height, seat depth, seat width and hand rest height) were measured using the anthropometric kit made up of metal rods. The measurements were than list out to see the difference between the body dimensions and the toilet chair dimensions which were causing accidents among old age people.

Results and Discussion

The anthropometric measurements of third age people were reported in Table 1. In this study toilet chairs were measured in relation to the respondent's anthropometric measurements. For designing any product ergonomically the measurements should be taken on the bases of percentile values, like for example for height 5th percentile should be taken or if possible than 50th and 95th percentile also, so that, different height people can be adjusted easily. For seat width 95th percentile and for seat depth 5th percentile value should be used. The products available in the local market were not designed by considering the percentile values that is why they were not found suitable by the target group. It can better seen by the Table 1, that there was a great mismatch between seat height and popliteal height, seat depth and buttock popliteal length, seat width and hip breadth, backrest height and sitting shoulder height, hand rest height and elbow rest height of the people of third age.

The dimensions of toilet chair given in Table 2 and Figure 1 depict that there was a great mismatch between the dimensions of locally available toilet chair and the ergonomically designed toilet chair. When the same was calculated statistically than it was found that there was a significant difference between the dimensions of both kinds of toilet chair. Locally available toilet chair is light in weight as comparison to ergonomically designed toilet chair that is also one of the reason of accidents as it was not good in maintaining the balance and slip easily during standing after sitting.

Locally Available Toilet Chair

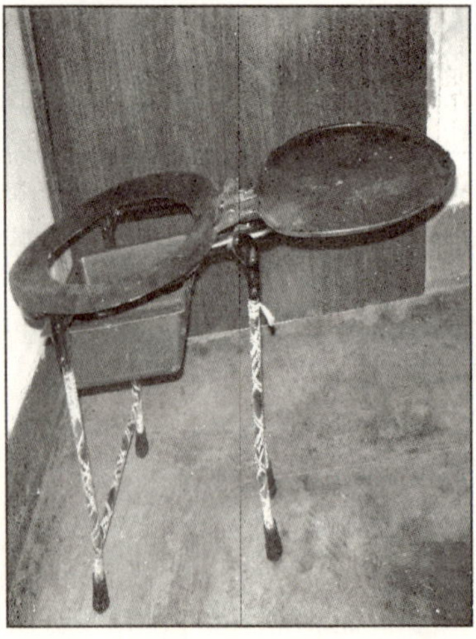

Ergonomically Designed Toilet Chair

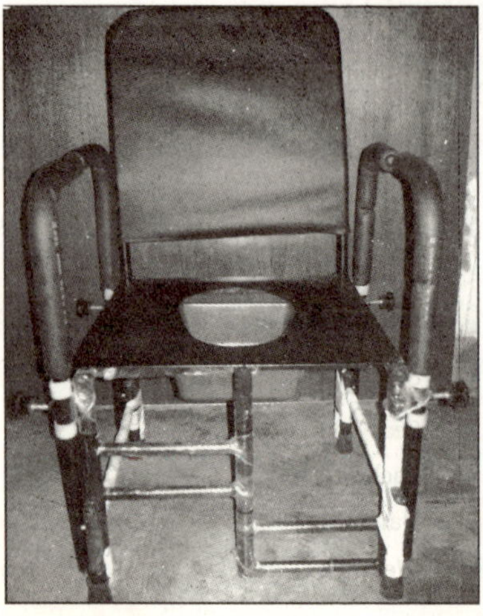

Figure 1 *Mismatch between Both Kinds of Toilet Chair*

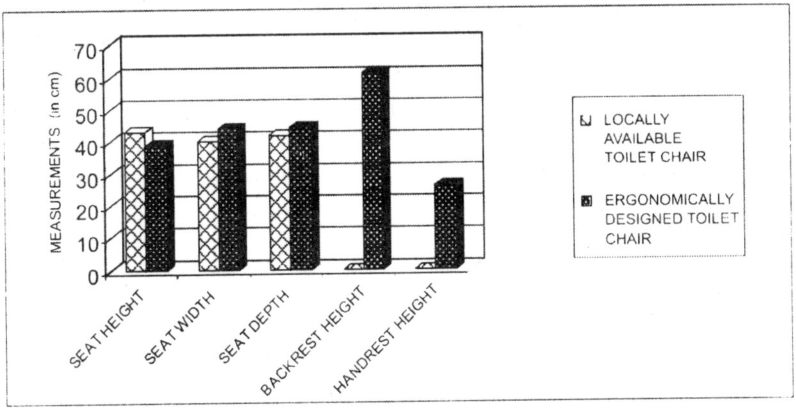

Table 1 *Comparison between Anthropometric Measurements and Chair Dimensions*

Sitting Measurements (cm)		*Measurements for Locally Available Toilet Chair (cm)*		*Measurements for Ergonomically Designed Toilet Chair (cm)*	
Sitting Shoulder Height	(61)	Backrest Height	(NP)	Backrest Height	(61)
Buttock Popliteal Length	(44.5)	Seat Depth	(42)	Seat Depth	(44.5)
Popliteal Height	(39)	Seat Height	(43)	Seat Height	(39)
Elbow Rest Height	(26)	Handrest Height	(NP)	Handrest Height	(26)
Hip Breadth	(44)	Seat Width	(40)	Seat Width	(44)

NP–Not Present.

Table 2 *Comparison between the Dimensions of Locally Available Toilet Chair and Ergonomically Designed Toilet Chair*

Measurements	*Locally Available Toilet Chair*	*Ergonomic Toilet Chair*	*Fishers t-value*
Seat Height*	43	39	3.951
Seat Width*	40	44	3.360
Seat Depth	42	44.5	2.100
Back rest Height*	NP	61	35.218
Hand rest Height*	NP	26	30.0322
Weight*	2.5 kg	10 kg	3.854

NP=Not Present * significant difference.

Conclusion

So, it is clear from the table as well as figure that there is a great mismatch between the locally available toilet chair and ergonomically designed toilet chair which was designed on the bases of the dimensions of third age people. So it is our duty that we should take care of our third age people about their limitations and try to provide them the products which will help them in easy going task and should not cause trouble to them.

References

Kinsella, K. and V.A. Velkoff. (2001) *An Ageing World: 2001*. U.S. Census Bureau, Series P95/01–1, US Government Printing Office, Washington DC.

U.S. Bureau of the Census. (1996) Population Projections of the United State by Age, Sex, Race and Hispanic Origin: 1995–2050. Current Population Reports, US Government Printing Office, Washington DC, pp. 25–1130.

14

Old Age Homes of Baroda

First Hand Encounter

RAMESHWARI PANDYA

The aim of home science, extension and communication is to keep an individual to get along with the changing world and to cope up with the modern ways of living. Thus, it is clear that home science extension and communication is not only concerned with intellectual development but also development of other traits which could help an individual to adjust and perform well in an environment which has important components as social, cultural as well as intellectual components. The main purpose of fieldwork programme is to sensitize and train students to contribute towards social change. Fieldwork offers students the opportunity to apply and translate theoretical knowledge into practice. The underlying philosophy of the programme is to sensitize students, to relevant macro level consideration by working closely at the micro level with the household and community in collaboration with various agencies and institution. The course fieldwork gives good learning experience and develops the ability to communicate effectively with people in the community.

Extension education forms a life contact between knowledge sources (institution) and social situation (community) by ways of addressing the problems and needs, extension education has to be broad and varied in its meaning to meet the interest of the people it serves. Swanson and Clarr (2000) connotes that "extension is an educational process which has its goals and the communication of useful information to people, then helping them to learn how to use it to build a better life for themselves, their families and their communities".

Extension services offer dynamic programmes keeping pace with the constantly changing conditions, as this field is the one, which stretch and reach out to the needy. In this case the elderlies are the most vulnerable members of the society. The students of the department are trained to become instructors and help in promotion of developmental communication messages and awareness programmes.

This chapter is based on the fieldwork, which was conducted under the course "Adult and Non-Formal Education" by the M.Sc. students of the Department of Extension and Communication, Faculty of Family and Community Sciences, Baroda of 2006–07 and 2007–08 batches.

The objectives of the Life Long Education Programme were:

1. To conduct activities on the basis of the needs and interests of the elderlies living in the old age homes and impart non-formal education.
2. To gain practical first-hand experience and sensitize students to the life of elderlies. Fieldwork was done in the following two old age homes:
   (i) Jalaram Seva Samaj Trust, Nizampura.
   (ii) Swami Premdas Jalaram, Warasia.

Methodology

The methodology is divided into

1. Construction of Tool.
2. Planning and Implementation of Activities.

Construction of the Tool

1. A questionnaire for data collection was developed and the questionnaire was divided in to sections:

Section I	• Profile of the elderly.
	• Background information.
Section II	• Perception of the elderly regarding the service provided at the old age home.

Data collection was done using interview schedule as well as observation schedule.

Planning of Activities

Planning is an inevitable step for any programme. All the planned activities should be very easy for the elderly so that they could easily participate. The activities were planned on the basis of the needs and interest of the elderly. Some entertaining activities were also planned like Antakshari, Bhajan so as to maintain their interest. Playing indoor games which were easy to participate for the elderlies were also selected.

Activities		
• Successful Ageing	• Mudra Session • Games (Passing the Parcel)	• Art of Living • Laughing Session • Acupressure
• Tips for decreasing depression	• Bhajan	• Garba • Drama
	• Religious Discourse	• General Tips for Health • Spiritual Talk
	• Yoga • Game (Object Identification)	• Science of old age • Stress Management • *Bhavi*

Different methods and materials ware used for the programme. Various teaching aids like charts, posters, flash cards, flip charts, board games were prepared and used during the fieldwork.

Old Age?

Old age consist of age nearing or surpassing average life span of human being, and thus end of human life cycle. Ageing cannot be exactly defined because it does not have same meaning in all the societies. In many parts of the world, people are considered old because of certain changes in their social roles or activities e.g. people may be considered old when they become grandparents or when they begin to do less or different work. In general ageing is seen in two ways: An orderly and regularly process of change, i.e., a gradual accelerating decline in the speed and precision of motor performances and of learning and immediate recall. The somatic musculature begins to fatigue more easily and to recover more slowly after exertion (Cameron, 1945).

On the other hand, ageing is seen as irregular, as a period of 'subtle variation'. It is not a simple slope which everyone slides down at the same speed. It is the flight of irregular stairs, down which some journey more quickly than another progress may be hastened or retarded by many factor such as heredity, diseases, environment or past habits (Howell, 1953: 45).

In the traditional Indian society, the elderly were holding positions of supremacy in the family and society endowed with special privileges. It is conventionally believed that wisdom will blossom with advancing age and hence, the elder with diversified rich life experiences would be in a better position to guide the younger generation in multifarious matters. In traditional Indian culture, old age is considered as one of the stages of human development wherein a person attains wisdom, maturity, social and economic stability with social recognition and emotional fulfilment leading to the last phase of life which is considered to be of spiritual salvation. Further, the elderly were the most respected in the family and centre of authority. All the decisions pertaining to the family were mostly made by them. They were also enjoying good respect in the society.

The situation, however, is fast changing because of the effect of rapid industrialization, urbanization and population pressure in the family. As a result of modernization, the family pattern is changing from joint and extended family to nuclear family. This has increased the problems of elderly because of prevailing family responsibilities and sometimes having no one to look after them due to migration of their grown up children.

The social aspects of old age are influenced by the relationship of the physiological effects of ageing and the collective experiences and shared values of that generation to the particular organization of the society in which it exists. In general the social status of an age group is related to its effective influence in its society/which is associated with that group's function in productivity. In agrarian societies the elderlies have a status of respectability. Their life experiences and knowledge are regarded as valuable, especially in preliterate societies where knowledge is orally transmitted. The range of activities in these societies allows the elderly to continue to be productive members of their communities. Familial relationships tend to be the focus of the elderly attention. However, as the family structure in industrialized countries has changed in the past few years from a unit encompassing several generations living in close proximity to self-contained nuclear families of only parents and young children, older people have become isolated from young generation. This has caused several problems to name few are psychological and ill health problems.

Psychological and Health Problems of the Elderly

All human beings advance in age and become old and it brings with it several changes. Because one reaches old age the psychological system become increasingly less efficient and less resistant to disease. Consequently the individual undergoes sufferings. There is a general belief prevailing in our society that illness as a part of being old. Psychological well-being is an important aspect of health. Like other human beings, elderly also have various psychological problems like memory impairment, depression, sleeplessness, fear, anxiety, social adjustment, insecurity, etc. These problems may be due to physiological as well as social factors. Cognitive impairment may cause functional problems for the older people. The physiological effects of ageing differ widely among individuals. However, chronic ailments, especially aches and pains, are more prevalent than acute ailments, requiring older people to spend more time and money on medical problems than younger people. Many elderly adults face significant life changes and stressors that put them at risk for depression. Those at the highest risk include older adults with a personal or family history of depression, failing health, substance abuse problems, or inadequate social support.

Causes and risk factors that contribute to psychological problems in the elderly include:

- *Loneliness and isolation*: Living alone; a dwindling social circle due to deaths or relocation; decreased mobility due to illness or loss of privileges.
- *Reduced sense of purpose:* Feelings of purposelessness or loss of identity due to retirement or physical limitations on activities.

- *Health problems:* Illness and disability; chronic or severe pain; cognitive decline; damage to body image due to surgery or disease.
- *Medications:* Many prescription medications can trigger or exacerbate depression.
- *Fears:* Fear of death or dying; anxiety over financial problems or health issues.
- *Recent bereavement:* The death of friends, family members, and pets; the loss of a spouse or partner.

The factors that precipitate emotional problems are loneliness, poor health, and loss of income, death of a spouse or close friend. Any one of these causes can lead to depression. It is known fact that depression are in the order of preoccupation with health, social inactiveness, helplessness, lack of interest sadness, lack of sleep or over sleep, self-pity, loneliness, lack of appetite and boredom are very common problems. The rising cost of medical care has caused a growing concern among older people and societies, in general resulting in constant revaluation and reform of institutions and programmes designed to aid the elderly with these expenses. Certain aspects of sensory and perceptual skills, muscular strength, and certain kinds of memory tend to diminish with age, rendering older people unsuitable for some activities.

Need for Old Age Homes in Society

India is land of traditions, customs and rich culture. We were known for our respect and love for elders. Parent-child relationship bond is considered most sacred in India. When a child enters school, the first thing he is taught is the verse from Taittiriya Upanishad that says, "*Matru devo bhava, Pitru devo bhava, Acharya devo bhava, Atithi devo bhava*" (Let you be one who worships mother, father, teachers and guests as God). This is something that everyone knows in India. Parents take lot of pains for bringing up their children and to help them to be in better position. In olden days, people used to live together in combined families. As per our culture, it is duty of the son to look after his parents. Now, the Indian society seems changing very fast and so also its moral values. Family structure has seen sea changes. Many people are not looking after their aged parents. Aged parents are either living alone or kept in old age homes. Everyone is in mad race of earning money, buying cars, going for foreign trips and they do not have time to spend with their parents and look after them.

Status of Old Age Homes in India

The dream of the people all over the world is to live long lives is now becoming a reality due to the socio-economic development of people and advancement in sciences, particularly medical sciences. In India about 7.5 per cent of the population is above 60 years and the life expectancy is increasing gradually. Old age was never a problem in India. Old age homes were alien concept and elder abuse was considered a Western problem. Not any more, as life expectancy has increased from 41 years in 1951 to 64 years today, hundreds of old age homes have sprung up in India. Neglect of parents has become a big issue, so much so that the Indian government has passed "The Maintenance and Welfare of Parents and Senior Citizens Bill 2006", which makes it imperative for adult children to look after their parents.

As of 1998, there were 728 old age homes in India. Detailed information about 547 of these is available. Out of these, 325 homes are free of cost while 95 old age homes are on pay and stay basis, 116 homes have both free as well as pay and stay facilities and 11 homes have no information. A total of 278 old age homes all over the country are available for the sick and 101 homes are exclusively for women.

As the role of families as a social safety net for the elderly is fast eroding, the poor among the elderly have become the most vulnerable sections of society in India. The Indian government is waking up to meet this challenge head on. At present over 500 NGOs are given grant-in-aid to provide services like old age homes, day care centres, medical facilities, etc., for the aged. The Delhi-based International Federation on Ageing has been campaigning for free health care for senior citizens; decrease in the age limit for pension; a bigger, respectable living allowance; change in the eligibility criteria so that even if the combined family income is Rs 8,000 the senior citizen is entitled to pension, creation and implementation of a social security scheme and so on.

We all will agree that old age homes are a necessity in the present-day scenario as the younger generation do not have the time or in many cases the resources to meet their needs (like medical expenses, special food, etc.). But old age homes should be considered only as a secondary option. Elders in the family are definitely an asset. It is they who can impart the much needed ethical values and code of conduct in the younger generation. Old age homes as an option should be considered only for the betterment of the senior citizens by way of better physical and mental status, greater possibility for social bonding, etc. Under no pretext should the aged be made to feel that they are a burden and hence turned away. Builders can also consider allocating a few houses for the senior citizens within an integrated township (at subsidized rates), so that the feeling of isolation goes away while proximity to dear ones is maintained.

Jalaram Seva Samaj Trust, Nizampura

Old age leads to retirement from occupation, physical/mental disabilities decrease in activities and a feelings conventional void in life. Due to family circumstances the desire to live last days in peace and harmony among one's near and dear one is left unfulfilled. The perceived actual decline in feelings of one's own, curt and even rude behaviour on the part of family members makes one feel dependent on others, leading future to decline in the zest of life. Life appears to be a burden due to dependency. The problem of living for rest of one's life in such a condition looks large and heavy by the ages. Society and government neglect the ages and what little is done is not enough. The aged, in this situation seek support. The presence of the elderly in a family, which led to a sense of discipline, peace and pleasure, in these days, is unwelcome. Wherever the fault may lie, the problem is commonly felt and a societal solution is called for. An attempt in the direction was made by some philanthropists of Vadodara believing in the maxim "Service to People is Service to God". They got together on the initiative of late Shri R.C. Gandhi, late Shri Kamlashankar Pandya and Shri J.D. Ray.

In August 1984 with the number of aged being only 7 (since increased to 20 by 1997 to 52 at present) an Old Age Home was started in a house of Navjivan Society, Ajwa Road. Shri J.D. Ray had allowed the use of a house owned by him for three years without charging any rent. It was at a location that was away from the city and there were logistic problems. Late Shri R.C. Gandhi arranged food from Hotel Express to be delivered; subsequently a helpful couple living nearby took on this responsibility. Late Shri R.C. Gandhi and his wife Smt Nirmalaben Gandhi donated Rs 5 lakh which gave birth to the Jalaram Seva Samaj Trust. A house at 13, Ashapuri Society was purchased and the home was shifted there, located well within the city. With increasing strength, it was once again shifted to Jalaram Seva Sadan, Nizampura.

A timetable has been set from morning till evening to occupy the aged at the present premises. Morning tea, lunch, afternoon tea and dinner are served. All except the ailing or disabled take meals together which fosters togetherness. For the ailing or disabled, room service is provided. Individual taste is catered to the extent possible. Care is being taken to provide a balanced diet. Jalaram Sevashram Trust provides food gains and grocery. As far as activities go, prayers in the morning and evening, religious discourses, bhajan singings, etc., are arranged regularly. Religious festivals are celebrated zestfully. Some eminent people are also invited from time to time for sharing their knowledge and experience.

Changes in lifestyle of the younger generation have made the creation of old age homes, a necessity. Instead of being laggards in the way of the fast moving youngsters, old age homes provide a space for the older generation to live life at their own peace and by their own terms. A nominal amount is charged from them. The advantage in an old age home is that is amongst one's peaces who understand each other better. With dissociation of different kinds, they can pool their abilities and be complementary to each other. When the ages stay with the young, the level of mutual understanding is less and not much complementary. Help, largely becomes a one-way street.

Health care is provided by Positive Health Clinic—a homeopathic institution run by Dr Mukesh Batra. Regular diagnostic camps are organized periodically with the help of S.S.G. Hospital and Yogini Vasantidevi Hospital, Vadodara. Shri Shashikant Sakarlal Velani, takes care of medical expenses.

The present status of the Jalaram Seva Samaj Trust is that there are 50 double rooms attached with bathroom and toilets. The resident has to pay Rs 600 per month for one year. Now, there are 14 couples and 65 elderly in the old age home who are from Vadodara, Mumbai, Saurashtra, etc.

Social Aspects of Senior Citizens Living at Jalaram Seva Trust

Table 1 *Table Showing the Senior Citizens in the Old Age Home*

(N=61)

Sex	*No*	*Percentage (%)*
Females	32	52.46
Males	29	47.54

The above table shows that there are about 53 per cent females and 47 per cent males in the old age home. The number of females is more than males.

Table 2 *Table Showing the Religion of Senior Citizens in the Old Age Home*

(N=61)

Religion	*No.*	*Percentage (%)*
Hindu	61	100

All the senior citizens in the old age home are Hindu by religion.

Table 3 *Table Showing the Time Duration of Senior Citizens in the Old Age Home*

(N=61)

Time Duration	*No.*	*Percentage*
0 years–3 years	32	52.46
3 years–6 years	18	29.51
6 years–9 years	11	18.03

The above table depicts that nearly half of senior citizens are living in the old age home for less than three years. It also reveals that only 18 per cent senior citizens live in the old age home for more than 6–9 years.

Table 4 *Table Showing the Age of Senior Citizens in the Old Age Home*

(N=61)

Age	*No.*	*Percentage (%)*
Below 50 years	3	04.92
51 years–60 years	6	09.84
61 years–70 years	21	34.43
71 years–80 years	21	34.43
81 years–90 years	8	13.11
Above 90 years	2	03.28

The above table reveals that equal percentage of senior citizens fall in the age group of 61–70 years and 71–80 years (34.43%). It is surprising that 3 per cent of senior citizens have crossed the age of 90 years.

Table 5 *Table Showing the Previous Residential Place of Senior Citizens in the Old Age Home*

(N=61)

Place	*No.*	*Percentage (%)*
Vadodara	49	80.33
Mumbai	5	08.20
Surat	3	04.92
Ahmedabad	1	01.64
Anand	1	01.64
Rajkot	1	01.64
Surendranagar	1	01.64

The above table shows that majority (80%) of senior citizens are from Vadodara city. Very less percentage, i.e., 8 and 5 have come from Mumbai and Surat respectively. There are senior citizens who have come from Ahmedabad, Anand, Rajkot and Surendranagar.

All the above tables show that people of different age and sex reside in the old age home. In this old age home there also lives a couple with their son who works in the kitchen.

Swami Premdas Jalaram Hospital, Warasiya

Swami Premdas elder's home is attached with the Premdas Jalaram Hospital. This is, a socio-economic organization, striving for the welfare of poor, needy and women and welfare to aged for last 20 years with the motto of 'be happy by making others happy', 'believing in peace' harmony and 'respect for all religious'. It believes 'service to mankind is worship to God'. Swami Premdasji was eleventh head (Mahant of spiritual, religious and social mission) in Sindh Pakistan. The principles were simplicity and service, purity and prayer. He was running charitable free dispensary in his village which served not only the place of his living, but even people from many other villages could take advantage of the free treatment and remained healthy and happy. Many mentally retarded people could regain their mental faculties by the medicines and blessings of Swamiji and many chronic patients could regain their lives by the treatment of swamiji. After partition of India, swamiji first came in Vrindaban in the year 1948. He constructed one good ashram 'TULSI NIVAS' in Vrindaban. In the year 1953 he got settled in Baroda. He believed that service to mankind is the real worship of God. Later on under his blessings and matured guidance, in 1988 Swami Premdas Seva Niketan was inaugurated with his sacred hands for rendering economic, educational, health and social services to the poor, need women, and aged. Hence, under Swami Premdas Seva Niketan Premdas Hospital, Medical Research Centre, Swami Premdas Elder's Home was started.

Objectives of the Institution

Swami Premdas Sewa Niketan mainly focuses on economic, educational, health and social services to the poor, needy women and aged. For the well-being of the neglected aged in the society, Swami Premdas Elder's Home was inaugurated with the objective of providing health and recreational facility to the elderly inmates, so that they could have good and comfortable stay and live with dignity and comfort.

Provision of Facilities

Swami Premdas Elder's Home is residential old age home which receives funds from the individual donors and also receives grant from social defence grant. The monthly charge for service and facility is Rs 650 per month. There are some criteria for admitting the elderly in to the old age home:

- The person should be 60 years and above.
- He/she should be self-dependant.
- He/she should be free from any kind of serious diseases.
- He/she should be able to take care of self.

Description of the Old Age Home

At present there are 25 inmates living in Jalaram Old Age home. The intake capacity of old age home is 30 as there are only 5 rooms available in which 6 persons can be accommodated. Couples cannot stay together as there are separate rooms for elderly men and elderly women. Bathrooms and toilet are common. There is one common hall in which all the recreational activities are conducted. As discussed earlier, the elder's home is attached with the Premdas Jalaram Hospital, all the medical care and expenses are taken care by the hospital itself. No extra charge is charged from the elderly inmates for medication. Regular health check-ups are organized. Yoga classes are conducted on the lawns of the old age home, daily from 6:30 am to 7:30 am for the elderly to maintain good health. Vegetarian nutritious food is served in the common dinning hall. Simple food like chapatti, sabji, rice and dal is served.

Findings and Observations

This section gives the details of the findings of the data which was collected with the help of questionnaire as well as case studies of elderly inmates.

Table 6 *Percentage Distribution of Elderly According to Sex*

(N=22)

Sex	*Percentage*
Male	63.63
Female	36.36

Table 6 shows that more than 63 per cent of the elderlies are male and less than 40 per cent of the elderlies (36.36%) are female.

Table 7 *Percentage Distribution of Elderly According to Age*

(N=22)

Sex	*Percentage*
Above 60 yrs	18.18
Above 70 yrs	54.54
Above 80 yrs	18.18
Above 90 yrs	9.09

Half of the elderlies are falling in the age group above 70. Equal percentage (18.18%) of the respondents are above 60 and above 80. Only 9.09 per cent falls under the age group of above 90.

Table 8 *Percentage Distribution of Elderly According to Religion*

(N=22)

Religion	*Percentage*
Hindu	86.36
Sindhi	13.63

Table 8 indicates that majority of the elderlies (86.36) were Hindu whereas very few (13.63%) were Sindhi.

Table 9 *Percentage Distribution of Elderly According to Marital Status*

(N=22)

Marital Status	*Percentage*
Married	18.18
Unmarried	43.07
Widow	36.37

Table 9 shows that more than 35 per cent of the elderly (36.37%) were widow and 31.09 per cent were widower, whereas less than 20 per cent of them (18.18%) were married and 13.07 per cent were unmarried.

Table 10 *Percentage Distribution of Elderly According to Education*

(N=22)

Educational Status	*Percentage*
Illiterate	12.5
Primary	50.0
Secondary	37.5

Table 10 indicates that 50 per cent of the elderly had schooling up to primary level education, whereas more than 35 per cent (37.5%) elderly had secondary level education. Very few of the elderly (12.5%) were illiterate.

Table 11 *Percentage Distribution of Elderly According to Type of Family*

(N-22)

Type of Family	*Percentage*
Joint family	25
Nuclear family	75

Table 11 indicates that majority of the elderly *(75%)* were from nuclear family whereas 25 per cent of the elderly were from joint family.

Table 12 *Percentage Distribution of Elderly According to Occupation*

(N=22)

Occupation	*Percentage*
Business	26.31
Service	36.84
Housewife	31.57
Unemployed	5.26

Table 12 indicates that more than 35 per cent (36.84%) of the elderly were doing services before coming to old age home whereas 31 per cent were housewives. More than 25 per cent (26.31) of the elderly were doing business and very few (5.26%) were unemployed.

Table 13 *Percentage Distribution of Elderly According to Duration of Living in Old Age Home*

(N=22)

Duration of Living in Old Age Home	*Percentage*
6 months to 12 months	23.52
1–5 years	52.94
6–10 years	5.88
11–15 years	10.52
16–20 years	5.88

More than half of the respondents (52.94%) were living in old age home for the last 1 to 5 years and less than 25 per cent (23.52%) were living since 6 to 12 months in old age home. Only 10 per cent (10.52%) of the elderly were living in old age home since 11 to 15 years, whereas very few percentage of the elderly (5.88%) were living in old age home since last 16 to 20 years.

Table 14 *Percentage Distribution of Elderly According to Reference for Coming in Old Age Home*

(N=22)

Reference For Old Age Home	*Percentage*
Self	47.36
Children	21.05
Relatives	26.31
Friends	5.26

Table 14 indicates that less than half of the elderly (47.36%) had come to the old age home by their own self and more than 25 per cent (26.31) had come by the reference of their relatives. About 21.05 per cent of the elderly had been referred by their children whereas only five per cent had been referred by friends. Elderly ladies were housewife. More than 20 per cent (26.31) of the elderly were doing business and very few (5.26%) were unemployed.

Table 15 *Percentage Distribution of the Elderly According to their Opinion on Following Point*

(N=22)

Better Place	*Percentage*
Old age home	61.53
Home	38.46

Majority of the respondent said that old age home is a better place of living whereas about 38 per cent said that home is better place for living.

Facilities for their Recreation

In the old age home following facilities are provided for their recreation and entertainment:

- Reading library/lending library, where they pass their time and gain knowledge and recreation.
- TV, radio and tape recorder are available for their recreation.
- Indoor games are played like antakshari, passing the parcel, etc.
- Periodically picnics are arranged to different religious places as well as priest gardens.
- Birthday celebrations are also arranged in nearby temples, where the monk of the temple garlands them, gives them flowers and blessings.
- Different festivals are also celebrated where feasts and gifts are given.
- Periodically religious discourses are arranged. Religious leader, philosophers, educationalists give educative, informative and positive information on health, nutritious food, which help them in their daily living.
- The elderly has to pay Rs 650 per month. They can pay it monthly in advance, whichever is favourable to them.
- Elderly are not getting breakfast from the old age home. They get lunch daily around 12:30 and get dinner around 7:30.
- Simple drinking water is provided, whereas cold water is provided for bathing. Only in the season of winter hot water is provided for bathing Water is available 24 hours.

- No special meeting place is available at the old age home. Elderly can meet their children guests either at individual room or in the common TV room.
- Female elderly have attached toilet facility in their room, whereas for males common toilet facility is provided.
- There are total five big rooms. In male's room accommodation is given to six persons whereas for females accommodation is given to three ladies.

Observations

Most of the elderly are interested in spiritual activities.

- They are eager to share their experiences whether happiness or bitterness of their life with others as they like to talk and they want somebody must listen.
- Some of them live in old age home by their own willingness.
- Few of them are not interested in participating in different activities.
- Few of them are interested in attending the programme but not able to participate in activities because of physical problems like less vision, pain in joints, etc.
- They reported that they do not get any chance to participate in any recreational activity from old age home and they wait eagerly for our visit.
- They have less mutual understanding and keep fighting among each other.
- The day when spiritual activities are organized many elderlies attend with lot of enthusiasm and interest.
- They are very enthusiastic to participate in games and they like to play indoor games.

Conclusion

Elderlies suffer from many problems like health, economic, social and emotional. They have performed their duties and responsibilities but now they are ignored by the people in our society. In spite of having abilities and capabilities at this age, they do not have any opportunities to utilize their time in a constructive manner. They have been tagged as helpless and simply burden for the family. As a result of all this they live a depressive life. They need some kind of encouragement to live healthy and happy life.

Although the establishment of various old age homes has helped these senior citizens to lead a healthy and secured life. In the old age homes they are well treated and they get a good opportunity to enjoy their life to the fullest. They get a familial environment and they can understand each other's problems very well. They feel better not because they are away from their children but that they get chance to express their feelings, ideas, thoughts, etc., with each other very freely.

Our journey to Jalaram Seva Trust and Premdas Trust was an enriching experience. We got to know the status of the senior citizens in these old age homes. They came from different background and lived together. We found that the programmes that we arranged for the senior citizens were successful. They enjoyed the recreational programmes. These types of programmes should be conducted for the senior citizens at a regular interval of time. Some recreational activity helps them to keep healthy and happy. They enjoy this and get motivated to live a happy life.

Paying gratitude towards senior citizens is not just a responsibility of an individual, an institution or any society but the responsibility rests on each and every citizen of our country. Senior citizens are the backbone of our building nation. They are the only one who have performed their duties and helped us to reach this era. We should never forget our obligatory role towards them. Then only the consistency of a developed nation can remain throughout this era.

Bibliography

Bond, John, P. Coleman and Sheila Peace. (1993) *Ageing in Society*. Sage Publications, New Delhi.

Cheney, W. (1996) *The Second Years*. Paragon House, New York, July.

Irudya Rajan, S., U.S. Mishra and P.S. Sharma. (1999) *India's Elderly: Burden or Challenge?* Sage Publications, New Delhi.

Kenny, R.A. (1982) *Ageing Process in Physiology of Ageing: A Synopsis*. Year Book Medical Publishers, London.

Kohli, A.S. (1996) *Social Situation of the Aged in India*. Anmol Publications Pvt. Ltd., New Delhi.

Ramamutri, P. (2004) *Indian Gerontology*. Serials Publications, New Delhi, January.

Rosow, Irving. (1967) *Social Integration of the Aged*. Free Press, New York.

Singh, R. (2005) *Health Psychology*. B.R. Publishing Corporation, Delhi.

Swanson and Clarr (2000) *Adult Education and Training in Extension*. Oxford University Press, New York.

Thara Bhai, L. (2002) *Ageing: Indian Perspective*. Decent Books, New Delhi.

Webliography

http://www.helpageindia.org/

http://www.whoindia.org/EN/Section20/Section26.htm

http://socialjustice.nic.in/social/sdcop/opersons.htm

http://india.gov.in/citizen/senior_citizen/policies_schemes.php

http://india.gov.in/citizen/senior_citizen_08.06.07/policies_schemes.php

http://www.webmed.com/

http://www.nios.ac.in/secpsycour/unit-14.pdf

15

Accidents Among Old Age People While Using Indian Toilet

NIRMAL KAUR AND PROMILA SHARMA

The world's older adult (60+ years) population is increasing by approximately 8,00,000 each month (Kinsella and Velkoff, 2001). Over the last decade, it has been clearly documented in worldwide population estimates that the average lifespan is increasing, as is the average age of the world's population (U.S. Bureau of the Census, 1996). During the past century the average life expectancy has increased by 28 years, from 45 to 73 years. This trend is expected to continue in the future. From the health policy point of view, it is of particular significance that the proportion of people aged 70 and above will increase by 40 per cent between 1995 and 2015. It can be assumed that the number of old people with disabilities will also rise, as any possible compression of morbidity would be too small to offset the effect of the rising numbers of older people in these populations.

Therefore, this age group should not be ignored in any ways and should be encouraged by the society and also helped in all ways so that they can live or survive easily in spite of having disabilities among them.

Objectives

1. To study the clinical history of the old age people.
2. To study the occurrence of accidents among old age people.

Methodology

In the present study descriptive design was planned to study the clinical history and occurrence of accidents among old age people. The present study was conducted in two regions of Uttarakhand state, i.e., Pantnagar and Rudrapur block of Udham Singh Nagar district. The whole list of families of Pantnagar and Rudrapur block was made who have old age people. Then out of that list the families were chosen randomly until the total sample size of 100 people each from both the blocks were selected. Now, there were 100 third age people from each block, out of which 50 per cent were male and 50 per cent were female selected. Thus altogether making total size of 200 people of old age may have accidental problems due to the use Indian toilet.

Result

When the clinical history of old age people was checked, then it was found that 42 per cent males and 62 per cent females were having joint problem. That is why only 59 per cent and 38 per cent males and females respectively, out of 100 males and 100 females were able to sit in squatting posture that is required in using Indian toilet.

Table 1 *Clinical History of the Respondents*

Criteria	*Male F=100*	*Female F=100*	*Total F=200*
Having joint problem	41 (41)	62 (62)	103 (51.5)
Able to sit in squatting posture	59 (59)	38 (38)	97 (48.5)
Problem in using Indian toilet	41 (41)	62 (62)	103 (51.5)
Type of problem in using Indian toilet:			
Pain in knee joints	41 (41)	62 (62)	103 (51.5)
Numbness in feet	28 (28)	32 (32)	60 (30)
Numbness in calf muscles	14 (14)	21 (21)	35 (18.5)
Standing after sitting	41 (41)	62 (62)	103 (51.5)
When feel pain:			
During standing	2 (2)	18 (18)	20 (10)
During sitting	—	—	—
All the time	—	42 (42)	42 (21)

Note: Figures in parentheses represent percentage.

Due to joint problem, the males (i.e., 39%) felt pain during walking whereas 42 per cent females felt pain all the time. Efforts were made to find out the problems in using Indian toilet and it was found that both the sexes were having pain in their joints and 28 and 14 per cent males and 32 and 21 per cent females had numbness in their feet and calf muscles, respectively, Whereas 41 per cent males and 62 per cent females also reported that they were having problem when they stand after using Indian toilet. They feel severe pain in their knees when they stand after sitting on Indian toilet. The cases of accidents listed in Table 2 also shows that 20.5 per cent males and 31 per cent females fall in their toilet during standing after sitting on Indian toilet.

Table 2 *Age and Sexwise Occurrence of Accidents*

Criteria	*60–65 yrs*		*65–70 yrs*		*Total*		*Chi-x^2 Values*
	M	*F*	*M*	*F*	*M*	*F*	
Fall due to standing after sitting	15 (15)	18 (18)	26 (26)	44 (44)	41 (20.5)	62 (31)	0.6466 NS
Fall due to no support	10 (10)	19 (19)	25 (25)	30 (30)	35 (17.5)	49 (24.5)	0.9404 NS
Fall due to slippery ness	4 (4)	7 (7)	8 (8)	11 (11)	12 (6)	18 (9)	0.0956 NS
Total	29	44	59	85	88	129	

Note: Figures in parentheses represent percentage.
NS—Not Significant.

Home injuries occur as a result of falls, slips and most of these accidents are considered preventable. Table 2 reveals age and sexwise distribution of total number of accidents among the people of third age. It was found that all accidents due to fall related to use of Indian toilet were more in case of females rather than males of third age, which results in injuries and it can be seen from the table that it was increasing with the increase in the age.

Conclusion

Thus we can see that due to the use of Indian toilet by the old age people, the chances of accidents are more because at this stage of life, joints problem is very common among them. Thus to avoid it, these people should be having the facility of either European toilet or if possible the specially made toilet chair for old age people should be used.

References

Kinsella, K. and V.A. Velkoff. (2001) *An Ageing World: 2001*. U.S. Census Bureau, Series P95/01-1, US Government Printing Office, Washington DC.

United Nations Population Division. (1999) World Population Prospects: The 1998 Revision. United Nations, New York.
www.popin.org/pop

U.S. Bureau of the Census. (1996) Population Projections of the United States by Age, Sex, Race and Hispanic Origin: 1995–2050. Current Population Reports, US Government Printing Office, Washington DC, pp. 25–1130.

16

Solitude in Old Age

URVASHI PANDE

The study examines the extent of solitude felt by the residents of an old age home in India where the family has always provided care and comfort to the elderly. A set of cultural norms backed by Hindu religious ideals has ensured the proper care of the elderly by the younger generation. It is often assumed that the absence of such a care system in old age homes may cause feelings of solitude and depression among the residents. The study, which is based on a study conducted in an old age home of Vallabh Vidya Nagar city in India, seeks to find out whether the loss of traditional social care does indeed create solitude and depression among the elderly. In the course of the study, few of the concepts were examined like involving solitude such as social isolation and desolation and seek to find out whether the experience of solitude of the residents of old age home can be understood within these conceptual frameworks.

Indian society provides a congenial set of conditions for a physically comfortable and emotionally satisfying old age. The extended family, which is the cornerstone of Indian social system, strong kinship ties and religious values extolling the virtues of old people have, for generations, acted as the natural social security for old people (D'Souza, 1982). The elderly never had to seek care and service outside the family and kinship group. This social security of the elderly flowed from their superior status in the family and by virtue of the fact the elderly parents enjoyed considerable authority and control in family matters, particularly over family property. This ensured their dominance in the family, and in turn, the children had to take care of their ageing parents as an obligation and as a sign of reverence.

But all this is changing. There has been a marked change in the treatment of the elderly compared to earlier periods. Many of the recent studies highlight the transition in the role and status of the elderly Indians from pre-industrial society to the existing industrial social order (D'Souza, 1982; Gangrade, 1999; Khan, 1997; Singh, 1999). Their main argument is that the elderly enjoyed a much higher status in pre-industrial society marked by group oriented social interaction, agricultural mode of production, extended family system, kinship and patriarchal authority. This, they contrast with the low position of the aged in the new industrial social order of India, affected by the processes of change such as modernization, industrialization, urbanization, secularization and changes in women's position.

In this kind of social situation, conflict and problems of adjustment have become a normal feature of the Indian families. Many of the elderly parents are compelled to leave their children and stay in old age homes. The old age homes, which were a rarity, have recently spread across the country, a fact that indicates the growing rift between the generations. It is a social expectation in India that the adult sons will take care of their aged parents and the daughters take charge of the parents in case the parents do not have sons (Vatuk, 1980; 1981; 1990). In case the sons stay separately from each other, the aged parents have to be under the care of one of the sons (Vatuk, 1981). It is sometimes asserted that the absence of any such care will cause adjustment problems, solitude and depression in the milieu of old age homes as the elderly persons are habituated to staying with their family members. The residents of the old age homes would find it difficult to adapt to the setting of the old age homes, which lacks the warmth and security of the family environment. There are some studies, which have indicated this factor of solitude and depression felt by the residents of old age homes. These studies (Mishra, 1993; Bagga, 1997; Dandekar, 1996; Nalini, 1997; Chadha and Kanwar, 1998; Irudya Rajan et al., 1999) have looked at the structure of old age homes, life of the inmates, their level of satisfaction or dissatisfaction, solitude, depression and family linkage of the inmates.

Analysing these studies, one finds that the majority of these studies have not looked at the dimension of solitude in details. It forms a minor aspect of their investigation of the lives of residents in the old age homes. Though Chadha and Kanwar (1998) compare the level of solitude between the institutionalized and non-institutionalized elderly using UCLA solitude scale, they do not provide details of causes of solitude, their subjective perception of feeling lonely and what strategies they employ to overcome it. Irudya Rajan et al's (1999) study indicates that the majority of the residents are 'overwhelmingly' happy, but it has not investigated what makes them feel so satisfied in the old age homes. Bagga's study (1997) mentions that the under-engaged and idle residents of old age homes feel more depressed and listless. Though she does not elaborate it, this is an interesting finding. It needs to be put in a perspective to understand its implications, which I attempt to do in this study.

In the light of these gaps in literature on solitude of residents of old age home, the study addresses the following questions. Do the elderly residents feel lonely and depressed in the old age home? If so, what are the main reasons for their solitude? If they do not feel lonely, what factors are responsible for it? Study will also investigate whether the residents of old age home are absorbed in activities in old age home. If they do, whether remaining in activity or work helps them in reducing solitude and enhances their self-esteem. It will also examine the concepts of social isolation and desolation to see if the feeling of solitude among the residents of old age home can be understood within this conceptual framework.

Concepts

Since the study focuses on the experience of solitude among the residents of old age home, it is essential to discuss the concepts of solitude. The concepts have been taken into account are 'social isolation', 'desolation', 'social solitude' and 'emotional solitude'.

Townsend distinguishes between social isolation and desolation in old age. Social isolation means having few contacts with family and community. Desolation means having an unwelcome feeling of lack or loss of companionship. It can be caused by the death or illness of the company of someone one loves. Townsend argues that though the two phenomena are related, it is desolation rather than isolation that cause solitude in old age (Bondevik and Skogstad, 1996). Absence or death of spouses is an indicator of desolation.

Townsend's distinction, somewhat, parallels Wiess' division of solitude into emotional solitude and social solitude (Russell et al., 1984). Emotional solitude results from the lack of a close, intimate attachment to another person. Those recently divorced or widowed may experience this form of solitude. On the other hand, social solitude is due to the lack of a network of social relationships in which the person is a part of a group of friends who share common interests and activities. Individuals who have recently moved to a new social environment (e.g., to a new city, job or college) may go through this type of solitude. Old persons who go to stay in a care institution, old age home or a nursing home may experience this form of solitude. While looking at the relationship between old age and solitude, researchers emphasize examining variables such as the available social contacts with significant others, like family members and friends, and the relationships between frequencies of contacts and desires for contacts (Bondevik and Skogstad, 1996). In this study I have examined if the residents suffer from desolation as mentioned by Townsend or go through social isolation as described by Weiss. The relationship of the elderly residents to their family members, friends at old age home and friendship developed with co-residents will reveal whether they suffer social isolation or not.

The activity theory of ageing propounds that engaging in some kind of activity or work facilitates old people to adjust to later years of their life and also helps them in avoiding solitude. Activity theory is essential a theory of successful ageing. It is based on the premise that the social and psychological health of a person is escalated by continued activity in a variety of roles. Havighurst who put forward this theory contends that there is a affirmative correlation between activity, mental and social adjustment. He holds that the role crisis created by retirement is overcome by engrossing new roles. He calls this role flexibiiity. He defines it as "the capacity of personal quality to change roles easily and increase or reduce activity" (Fennell et al., 1988). In other words, people cannot be cheerful unless they stay socially active. People, after retirement, try to fill in the vacant time by engaging in some kind of activity. It helps in maintaining mental and physical health of the old person. The present study examine whether remaining in activity has a positive correlation with reduction of solitude and increase in self-esteem of the elderly residents of old age homes.

Setting and Method

A semi-structured interview schedule was used to tap the respondents' experience of solitude, living condition in the old age home, life satisfaction and family linkage. The simple observation method to collect data on their daily schedule was used.

Results and Discussion

In the Anand Niketan Vruddhashram, where the study was conducted, the sex ratio of the respondents shows that out of the ten respondents, seven were males and three were females. The respondents belong to four age groups: five of the respondents are in the age group of seventy to seventy-four, two each in the age groups of sixty-five to sixty-nine and eighty and above and one person is in the age group of sixty to sixty-five. Thus, half of the respondents are concentrated in the age group of seventy to seventy-four. The findings also show that there are very few respondents who came here immediately after their retirement.

India, being a caste-based society, it is important to look at the caste background of the respondents. Six of the respondents are Brahmins and the rest four are in the other upper caste category. This shows that the old age home has predominantly upper caste residents.

The marital status of the respondents shows that four respondents are either widows or widowed. The rest six respondents have their spouses living, amongst whom three stay with their spouse at old age home and the spouses of the other three are at home with their children.

The data on number of children of respondents shows that four of the respondents have one to three children whereas rest six has four to six children. This finding suggests that the elderly residents had children who could take care of them.

The sources of income of the respondents reveal that eight of them meet their expenses from their pension. One respondent pays her expenses drawing on her deceased husband's pension. And, in the case of the other respondent, her husband takes care of the expenses.

The study revealed that six of the residents came from cities (Punjab, Hisar and Vallabh Vidya Nagar) and rest four respondents were from towns of Uttar Pradesh. The study conducted by Dandekar (1996) in old age homes of Maharashtra also confirms that the majority of the residents are usually from the cities and small towns. One can surmise that either the families in the villages take care of their aged members or the concept of old age homes has not yet gained momentum in the countryside.

The study further showed that the decisions of the elderly to reside in the old age home were influenced by multiple factors. Four of the respondents said that it was their disagreement and conflict with sons and daughters-in-law that forced them to come here. Another three reported maladjustment with the family members as a reason for leaving home. The thought of seeking spiritual development in later life drove three of them to this place. One respondent complained that since there was nobody to take care of her, she was compelled to reside in an old age home. It needs to be noted that most of the respondents felt that they found it uncomfortable to stay with their children. Their children did not have any time for them. They differed on many matters, which created an atmosphere of tension and uneasiness in the family. So they felt it was better to stay away from their families. Though many tried to justify their presence in the old age home, saying in old age, one should leave the family and devote the rest of the life to religious activities. For such activities, this old age home is ideally suited. However, subsequent probe questions revealed that 'self-unfoldment', as the Ashram management calls it, is not the driving force, rather it is maladjustment with the family members that brought them here. This finding is in line with the observations made by Mishra (1993), Nalini (1997), and Irudaya Rajan et al. (1999), that the elderly persons are opting to stay in old age homes to avoid conflict and domestic quarrels at home. Mishra (1993) mentioned in her study that the children of the elderly residents did not object to and expressed no sadness at the decision of their parents to reside in old age home. Rather they felt relieved. The elderly residents, however, felt that they had been driven out of the family.

The respondents were asked a series of questions on their experience and extent of solitude. All the respondents, barring one, expressed that they do not feel lonely and depressed in the environment of the old age home. In fact, they do not feel isolated from their family members or from their friends and acquaintances. They also do not miss the atmosphere of their homes. This finding goes against the studies made by Mishra (1993), Bagga (1997), Nalini (1997), Chadha and Kanwar (1998) that, in India, the residents of old age homes suffer from solitude, depression, isolation and health hazards. Mishra (1993) found that all the inmates felt dissatisfied residing in old age homes as they felt segregated from the family and the wider community. They all wanted to go back to their families to spend the rest of their lives with their near and dear ones.

Similarly Bagga (1997) in her study of all-female old age homes showed that younger entrants to the old age homes feel more depressed than their senior counterparts. Further, she added that the residents felt more lonely and depressed in old age homes where they stayed as guests and did not prepare food themselves. Chadha and Kanwar (1998) have also mentioned in their study that the institutionalized aged feel more lonely and depressed as they lack social network support and do not feel "the level of kinship" felt by non-institutionalized aged. My findings differ from these studies.

The respondents explained that they do not feel lonely because they are in constant touch with their family members. It was found that in case of half of the respondents, their children visit them once in one or two months. Sometimes they call up their parents and ask about their health. Even the residents themselves visit their children quite often. There are very few residents whose children visit them rarely or not at all. Thirty per cent of the respondents replied that both the parents and children visit each other whenever they feel like. Only one or two respondents expressed their inability to go home because of health and physical constraint. This shows that both the elderly residents and their children have not severed their relations with each other, though they found it difficult to stay together. Some of the respondents fondly remember their grandchildren and say that they feel very happy whenever they come to visit them. Sometimes they call up specifically to speak to their grandchildren. The constant contact with the family members is one of the factors why they do not feel social solitude. They also do not experience desolation.

Bondevik and Skogstad (1996) compared the experience of solitude between residents living in nursing homes and residents living in the community. Though they did not find any significant difference in the level of solitude between two groups, they reported that the residents in nursing homes with frequent contacts with family and friends experienced less solitude than the residents in nursing homes without such contacts. This factor is corroborated in this study. The residents in the old age home did not experience solitude because of their frequent contacts with family and friends. Chadha and Kanwar (1998) have also reported that the institutionalized elderly feel more lonely and depressed than their non-institutionalized counterparts because they had less social support at their behest.

Further, the respondents were found to be engaged in various tasks within the old age home. Half of the respondents help the

Ashram according to their capacities. For instance, one of the residents, who was a journalist, looks after the Ashram publications. Another, who was an accountant, helps in managing the Ashram accounts. He said, "I am retired but not tired." One female resident of the Ashram assists in the management of the Ashram. She also takes study classes on Yoga and other forms of meditation. All the residents of the Ashram attend the daily prayer sessions, meditation classes and sermons given by the religious guru, who heads the Ashram.

Seven of the respondents, who said that they do something or the other for the old age home, remarked that they felt satisfied doing some work for the Ashram. When they were asked whether engaging in activities, enhances their self-esteem, they answered in the affirmative. They also mentioned that being absorbed in various tasks in the old age home, helps them get rid of solitude. This finding corroborates the assumption of the activity theory that engaging in various roles, not only improves the physical and mental health of the elderly but also instils in them a sense of self-esteem. They do not form a negative opinion of themselves. As the study shows, the respondents do not think of themselves as useless or redundant. Rather, participation in the tasks of the Ashram imparts a feeling of self-fulfilment to them. They feel that they are not only capable of taking care of themselves but can also contribute to the management of the old age home. This study thus shows that engaging in activities have a positive influence on the mental health of the residents.

The respondents were asked about their relationship with other residents. Six respondents said they have very good relationship with co-residents. The rest four described their relationship as friendly. Overall, they have developed a bond of friendship with the fellow residents, which is also instrumental in reducing their solitude. When they were asked how they felt about their life in the old age home, six respondents replied that they are highly satisfied with their life at old age home. Another three described their life as satisfactory. Only one person said that she is partially satisfied. To sum up, it appears that they lead quite a satisfactory and peaceful life at the old age home. To a series of questions on the comparison of life between their homes and the old age home, eight of the respondents felt they are happier here at the old age home. Only one person replied he felt equally happy at home and at the old age home. All, barring one, felt that their health had improved after coming to the old age home.

Their satisfaction with the life in the old age home is not surprising as the factors such as regular contact with their family members, participation in the daily schedule of the Ashram, engagement in the activities of the Ashram and a positive relationship with the fellow residents have made their stay comfortable. They do not feel isolated from their family and do not suffer from experience of solitude and depression.

Another major reason why they do not feel lonely and try to engage themselves in the activities of the old age home is the influence of the religious teachings. The old age home, being run by a religious organization, has scheduled the daily routine with a series of religious activities such as prayer sessions, meditation and sermons. In the sermons, the residents are told about the duties of an elderly parent as laid down in the Hindu scriptures.

The Hindu system talks of four stages of life of which last two stages pertain to old age. These two stages of life cycle are marked by dissociation from worldly activities and retirement to forest where spiritual orientation is cultivated in pursuit of salvation after death (Kapadia, 1966). Though these stages of life are not strictly adhered to, nevertheless, they are of utmost significance in influencing the life pattern of the aged. As the concept of setting off for spiritual pursuit to the forest does not have any takers in contemporary India, certain religious organizations build homes, where old people can stay and devote to their lives to God. Here they are asked to minimize their family contacts and friends circle.

The Anand Niketan Vrudhashram does inculcate this religious teaching among the residents. The residents are made to understand the idea of living alone and engaging in religious activities. This factor goes a long way in making the residents adjust to the situation at the old age home. Bondevik and Skogstad (2000) in their study on oldest-old in Bergen found no significant correlation between solitude and religiousness. Though, the majority of the respondents reported that religion was important to them, no connection could be established between the two. But my study suggests that the religious teachings of Hinduism regarding attitude in old age and its partial practice among the residents of the old age home have helped in overcoming solitude to a great extent. I describe it as a partial practice because the older persons do not go to forest to contemplate on spiritual matters and do not sever all contacts with family members. They stay in the old age home, retaining contact with the family members, while at the same time observing religious practices. This is perhaps similar to what Paul Hiebert (1981) terms "mental mendicancy" in his study of the Hindus in Konduru village of Andhra Pradesh. He found that the villagers did not strictly follow the scriptural ideals but reinterpreted it in the sense that a section of the villagers chose the path of abstract meditation at home surrounded by family members, arguing that detachment is possible in any situation and context.

Hence the peculiar and unique nature of the old age home with its emphasis on engagement in various activities and stress on partial disengagement from family responsibilities are instrumental in facilitating a satisfactory stay of the residents of the old age home.

Conclusion

In this study, it has been argued that the residents of the old age home do not feel lonely and depressed being away from home. They are quite satisfied with their life in the old age home and, even saying that they are happier here than at home. The residents do not experience either social isolation or desolation.

This is due to the regular mutual visits of the residents and family members and the effort on the part of the old age home officials and residents to engage themselves in various activities. Another factor, which is largely responsible for the adjustment of the residents to the old age home, is the preaching of the Hindu religious ideals that concerns old age. The Hindu scriptures lays down that the old parents must turn over the family responsibilities to their adult children and devote themselves to spiritual matters. In the old age home, the residents are made to realize through sermons that they should not feel lonely and crave for the presence of family and friends, but engage in religious activities and any other work that interests them.

While examining the activity theory of ageing, which holds that remaining in activity has a positive correlation with mental health and self-esteem of the elderly. The respondents in present study agreed that engagement in activities have bestowed them a feeling of self-reliance. They do not feel obsolete and redundant. It also helps them to get rid of solitude.

It is very difficult to arrive at a generalization from this study as it draws upon a small number of respondents. Since the study did not look at other types of old age homes such as old age homes run by voluntary agencies or old age homes managed by the government, it is not possible to generalize that elderly residents do not experience solitude in all old age homes in India.

The findings also differ from earlier studies, especially those which were carried out in other types of old age homes, particularly free old age homes where solitude was reported. It needs to be mentioned that the respondents in this study pay for their stay, which indicates a choice rather than a compulsion to reside in the old age home. This could be factor in getting a result that differs from earlier studies. Another important factor is perhaps the religious nature of the old age home.

Nonetheless, the findings point to a significant trend that needs to be taken up in further studies. It needs to be investigated if the presence of the same set of variables, such as regular contact with family and friends, good relationship with co-residents and absorption in work inside the old age home, facilitates in getting rid of solitude and depression among residents in old age homes other than of religious orientation. It would also be interesting to study whether residents of similar old age homes run by other religious organizations in India such as the Christians and Muslims, do manage to avoid solitude due to the influence of their religious tenets. The outcome of these studies would be particularly useful if they could suggest the right setting for the old age homes where the residents would truly feel at home.

References

Bagga, Amrita. (1997) "A Study of Women in Old Age Homes of Pune", in Indrani Chakravarty (ed.), *Life in Twilight Years*. Calcutta: Kwality Book Company, pp. 171–175.

Bondevik, M. and A. Skogstad. (1996) "Solitude among Oldest Old: A Comparison between Residents Living in Nursing Homes and Residents Living in the Community". *International Journal of Ageing and Human Development*, 43 (3): 181–197.

——. (2000) "Solitude, Religiousness, and Purpose in Life in the Oldest Old". *Journal of Religious Gerontology*, 11 (1): 5–21.

Chadha, N.K. and P. Kanwar. (1998) "Psychosocial Determinants of Institutionalised Elderly: An Empirical Study". *Indian Journal of Gerontology*, 12 (3 and 4): 27–39.

D'Souza, Victor. (1982) "Changing Social Scene and its Implications for the Aged", in K.G. Desai (ed.), *Ageing in India*. Bombay: TISS, pp. 71–79.

Dandekar, Kumudini. (1996) *Elderly in India*. New Delhi: Sage.

Fennell, G., C. Phillipson and H. Evers. (1988) *Sociology of Old Age*. Milton Keynes: Open University Press.

Gangrade, K.D. (1999) "Emerging Conception of Ageing in India: A Socio-cultural Perspective", in Arun Bali (ed.), *Understanding Greying People of India*. New Delhi: Inter-India Publications, pp. 36–57.

Hiebert, Paul. (1981) "Old Age in a South Indian Village", in Pamela Amoss and Steven Harrell (eds.), *Other Ways of Growing Old: Anthropological Perspectives.* Stanford: Stanford University Press, pp. 211–226.

Irudya Rajan, S. U.S. Mishra and P.S. Sarma. (1999) *India's Elderly: Burden or Challenge?* New Delhi: Sage.

Kapadia, K.M. (1966) *Marriage and Family in India*. Bombay: Oxford University Press.

Khan, I.H. (1997) "Reflections on Ageing in Indian Context", in M.G. Hussain (ed.), *Changing Indian Society and Status of the Aged.* New Delhi: Manak, pp. 59–72.

Mishra, Saraswati. (1993) "Scenario of Segregated Seniors: A Case Study of Inmates of Old Age Homes". *Indian Journal of Gerontology*, 7 (3 and 4): 104–110.

Nalini, B. (1997) "Institutional Care for the Aged: The Issues and Implications", in Indrani Chakravarty (ed.), *Life in Twilight Years*. New Delhi: Kwality Book Company, 1997, pp. 63–77.

Russell, D., C.E. Cutrona, J. Rose and K. Yurko. (1984) "Social and Emotional Solitude: An Examination of Weiss's Typology of Solitude". *Journal of Personality and Social Psychology*, 46 (6): 1313–1321.

Singh, Dalip. (1999) "Day Care Centres and Home for Aged", in Arun Bali (ed.), *Understanding Greying People of India.* New Delhi: Inter-India Publications, pp. 214–230.

Vatuk, Sylvia. (1980) "Withdrawal and Disengagement as a Cultural Response to Ageing in India", in Christine Fry (ed.), *Ageing in Culture and Society: Comparative Viewpoints.* Praeger: New York, pp. 126–148.

——. (1980) "Cultural Perspectives on Social Services for the Aged in India", in Charlotte Nusberg and Masako Osako (eds.), The Situation of the Asian/Pacific Elderly: Proceedings of Two Symposia held in Hong Kong and San Diego. Washington DC: International Federation on Ageing, pp. 98–109.

——. (1990) "'To be a Burden on Others': Dependency Anxiety among the Elderly in India", in Owen Lynch (ed.), *Divine Passions: The Social Construction of Emotion in India*. Berkeley: University of California Press, pp. 64–88.

17

Age-Defying Foods

VANISHA S. NAMBIAR

Diet contributes in many ways to the development of age related diseases. Undoubtedly, the earlier a healthy lifestyle, including an adequate nutritional intake is adopted—the better. The potential impact of dietary manipulation in the maintenance of physical and cognitive function between middle and old age has profound consequences for optimization of health, independence and well-being for later year. In fact, nutrition plays a very important role in the development of human resource.

Certain foods are essential for maintaining good health and nutrition in humans. Foods, particularly those of plant origin, contain a wide range of non-nutrient phytochemicals that are elaborated by plants for their own defence and other biological functions. Consumption of foods that slows the ageing process, such as those rich with vitamins and minerals can help in the reversal or reduction of the rate of body's ageing processes.

Phytochemicals present in plant foods have a useful role in prevention of chronic diseases such as cancer, diabetes, cardiovascular diseases, cataract and gallstones. These antioxidant rich foods help the body to fight against the free radicals (molecules which are destructive to the body, sometimes becoming carcinogenic, and speeden up the ageing process). Such foods that have disease preventing potential are designated as 'functional foods'. These have been categorized in various categories such as enhancers of body immune system; preventers of diabetes and heart diseases;

hypocholoesterolaemic agents; promoters of digestion and absorption and retardants of ageing.

Consideration is now given to the potential benefit of antioxidant micronutrients and phytochemicals in order to support the scientific evidence behind the almost universal dietary guideline: "*eat plenty of vegetables (including legumes) and fruit*".

Foods that Affect the Brain

Ageing of the brain is generally caused by an increase in oxidative stress. Several studies have shown that oxidative damage to the mitochondria (the furnace of the cell) and to the DNA of the brain cell can lead to malfunction or even death of these very sensitive brain cells. In medical terms this leads to loss of cognition. In lay man's term there is a decrease in our ability to think or reason. Ageing of brain is essentially the first stage of degeneration of these very important cells in our body. Diseases such as Parkinson's or Alzheimer's disease represent the end stages of oxidative damage to the brain.

A number of studies have suggested that dietary intervention with various nutrients may help to delay the progression of age-related mental deterioration. The potential effect of certain vitamins and minerals in the prevention and delayed progression of many age-related chronic diseases is largely due to their ability to either prevent the formation of free radicals or to scavenge them once they are formed, either directly (e.g., Vitamin C, E and Beta-carotene) or indirectly (e.g., copper/zinc, superoxidedismutase, selenium-dependent glutathione peroxidase).

Table 1 *Nutrients/non-Nutrients that Affect the Brain*

Vitamin B complex especially B_{12}, B_6 and folate	Prevents hyperhomocysteinaemia, which has been suggested to represent a metabolic link in the pathogenesis of old age dementias.
Vitamin C and Vitamin E, selenium, Glutathione and N-acetyl–L-cysteine and zinc	Slow progression of early Parkinson's disease and Alzheimer's dementia
Vitamin E	Protects the brain and the peripheral nerve cells.

Cont'd...

Cont'd...

Vitamin C	Can concentrate in the tissue and fluid around the brain and nerves
Glutathione	Most important antioxidant within the brain and nerve cells (nutrients such as vitamin C, alpha-lipoic acid and CoQ_{10} help in regeneration of glutathione).
Alpha-lipoic acid	It can regenerate vitamin C, vitamin E, intracellular glutathione and CoQ10. It can attach itself to toxic metals in the brain and help eliminate them from the body.
Coenzyme Q_{10}	This is a very potent antioxidant as well as one of the most important nutrients for the production of energy within the cell (mitochondria).
Biogenic amines such as 5-hydroxy tryptamine, nonadrenaline, tryamine, dopamine and their precursors (bananas, tomatoes and avocados and in spices such as pepper)	These neuroactive chemicals have special effects on brain function, learning and behaviour and they sharpen mental agility.
Anemia caused by iron, Vitamin B_{12} or folate deficiency; Vitamin A deficiency and protein energy malnutrition	Can also cause an impairment of mental function.

Age-Related Macular Degeneration

Quality of vision and appetite has been shown to be positive, independent and significant predictors of energy and nutrient intake in a high risk group of elderly. Age-related macular degeneration (AMD) is the leading cause of blindness among elderly in the developed world. Populations with a high lutein and zeaxanthin intake have shown a significantly lower risk of AMD compared to those in the lowest quintile of intake.

Lycopene is responsible for the red colour in tomatoes, water-melon, pink grapefruit, guava and a limited number of other foods. Lutein and zeaxanthin are carotenoids that are deep yellow in colour and are found abundantly in dark green leafy vegetables and in smaller amounts in other colourful fruits and vegetables, such as corn and capsicum. Lycopene intake is found to be protective against prostrate cancer. Mix fruits packed with vitamin A (peaches and apricots) and vitamin C (citrus fruits, strawberries and blueberries). With many options, these fruits are easy to work into a diet as snacks, side dishes or additions to salads. They are also an extremely healthy dessert for the elderly population.

Immunity

Some phytochemicals have the potency for augmenting both humoral and cell mediated immune function. Vitamin C rich foods such as citrous fruits, amla, guava, and carotenoids (green leafy vegetables, yellow, red and orange coloured fruits and vegetables) have beneficial effects on immune function, thereby reducing cancer risk by enhancing the tumour surveillance of the immune system. Foods containing antioxidants help the body fight free radicals. These molecules are destructive to the body, sometimes becoming carcinogenic. They take a toll on the body, speeding the ageing process. Eating antioxidant-rich foods regularly helps you decrease the damage caused by free radicals in the body. Cruciferous vegetables including cabbage and cauliflower can help prevent cancer and stave off heart disease.

Dietary Guidelines for Older People

1. Enjoy a wide variety of nutritious foods.
2. Keep active to maintain muscle strength and a healthy body weight.
3. Eat at least three meals a day.
4. Dietary fibre should be around 25–40 gram/day. Preferred fibre is soluble fibre coming from oats, beans, legumes, vegetables and fruits
5. Care for your food: prepare and store it correctly.
6. Eat plenty of vegetables (including legumes) and fruit.
7. Eat plenty of cereal, bread and pastas.
8. Eat a diet low in saturated fat. Total fat intake should be between 15–30 per cent of total calories which amounts to about 50 gram/day in an average diet of an adult. This is both visible fat used for cooking and invisible fat already present in foods. It is best to include low fat foods. Use combination of oils for different food preparation/blended oils.
9. Drink adequate amounts of water and/or other fluids.
10. If you drink alcohol, limit your intake.
11. Choose foods low in salt and use salt sparingly.
12. Use added sugars in moderation.

Foods that Increase Longevity/Age-Defying

1. *Avocado:* This is one of the most alkalizing foods available. Avocados are very high in vitamin E which is essential for glowing skin and shining hair. It also help keeps those wrinkles off your face. Have a raw avocado salad or a steamed one with some salt to add effect.
2. *Berries:* All berries, especially gooseberries, are very rich in vitamin C and therefore highly useful to the body. Vitamin C helps in proper blood circulation and provides minerals and salts to all the body parts. Needless to say this helps the body to fight against ageing and keep fit.
3. *Green vegetables:* Broccoli, spinach, lettuce, salad leaves and other such greens are highly beneficial for the body. Not only do they help keep the body weight low but also help fight toxins. Fighting toxins is important because a highly toxic body is like a magnet for all kinds of diseases that can harm the body.
4. *Garlic:* This is one of the most important foods provided to us by nature. The benefits of garlic are numerous. It helps prevent cell degeneration, helps keep the blood thin and also prevents heart diseases. It is most beneficial when eaten raw.
5. *Ginger:* This root facilitates digestion and is therefore essential for the body. Ginger keeps bowel movement in shape, thereby enabling good gut health.
6. *Nuts:* Almonds and cashew nuts are like power houses of energy. Consuming nuts on a daily basis will fight that lethargic feeling and fill the body with immense energy.
7. *Yogurt:* Yogurt is rich in important minerals like potassium, calcium, protein and B vitamins. Apart from these, what makes yogurt one of the most powerful foods is the presence of live bacteria in it. This bacteria helps absorption of nutrients in the intestines and stabilizes the immune system, which is a necessity for the aged.
8. *Whole wheat pasta and brown rice:* Carbohydrates are long term energy foods and should never be given up unless you want to invite trouble. Substitute white pasta and rice with whole wheat pasta and brown rice and you will instantly feel the difference in your energy level.
9. *Melons:* Watermelons and musk melons not only have an alkalizing effect on the body but also provide the body with essential fluids that it needs for performing various tasks.

10. *Water:* Nothing compares to water. Stay away from those aerated drinks for it takes 32 glasses of water to balance out the ill effects of one glass of soda. Water is essential for our body. It flushes out all the toxins from the body. It also provides fluidity for the flow of blood. At least eight glasses of clean pure water must be consumed on a daily basis.

Age Accelerators

Over the previous three decades, Asian Indians have become more affluent and urbanized. These changes have resulted in higher consumption of calories, saturated fat, trans fat, simple sugars, carbohydrates and lower intake of fibre, MUFA and n–3 PUFA as compared to the years preceding the change.

There are certain foods which are likely to deteriorate the body functions. These foods such as red meat and full-fat dairy can cause premature wrinkling and lead to inflammation that slows brain function.

Fried and packaged foods often contain trans-fats that clogs arteries and pack on belly fat. Cooking oils and animal foods should be used in moderation and vanaspati/ghee/butter should be used only sparingly

Only minimal amount of oil should be used while cooking and no oil containing trans-fat (vanaspati); instead use a variety of oils in cooking.

Soda: The high fructose corn syrup in soda can weaken bones. The regular and diet drinks with soda contain phosphoric acid, a chemical that makes it harder for your bones to absorb calcium.

Cookies, cakes and white flour: refines carbohydrates boost your risk of age-related macular degeneration as well as contribute to weight gain.

Foods which usually cause degeneration and ageing are:

- High levels of carbohydrate.
- Sugar.
- Milk (especially homogenized milk) and cheese.
- Caffeine, including tea, coffee, chocolate, cola, chuppa chups.
- Chocolate (MUCH worse than you ever realized). However dark chocolates are hypocholesteronomic.
- Cigarettes.
- White flour.

- Microwaved food.
- Chemicals such as flouride (which is a rat poison).
- Artificial sweeteners (especially aspartame/nutrasweet).
- Alcohol.
- Processed foods with artificial colourings (as in Gatorade) /Additives/Monosodium glutamate (MSG).
- Preserved meat/moderate to high levels of meat/meat from animals on unnatural diets (e.g., pork).
- Margarine.
- Cottonseed oil.
- Hydrogenated oils/Oil that is not cold pressed/expeller pressed (use olive oil, butter or ghee).
- Deep fried foods/chips/French fries.
- Seafood which are garbage eaters (e.g., oysters).
- Foods with high levels of mercury. This includes most fish, such as tuna.
- Aluminium, especially from aluminium cookware.
- Genetically Modified Food (GMOs). At present, this is about 50 per cent of all soy and corn. Even organic soy and corn can have GMOs in it unless otherwise stated.

Health promotion activities, including changes in diet and exercise patterns, can contribute to an increase in life expectancy and better health. Such benefits are most effective when healthy lifestyles are adopted early in life, however, positive effects can occur at any age.

References

Hertog, M.G., E.J.M. Feskens, P.C.H. Hollmsn, M.B. Katan and D. Kromhout. (1999) "Dietary Antioxidant Flavanoids and the Risk of Coronary Heart Disease: Zulfan Study". *Lancet*, 342: 1007–1011.

Krishnaswamy, K. and N. Raghuramulu. (1998) "Bioactive Phytochemicals with Emphasis on Dietary Practices". *Ind J Med Res.*, 108: 167–181.

Mehta, P. and V.S. Nambiar. (1999) Ageing, Nutrition and Health. A Report based on the Proceedings of a National Conference, Department of Foods and Nutrition, M.S. University of Baroda.

Misra, A., P. Chowbey, B.M. Makkar, N.K. Vikram, J.S. Wasir, D. Chadha, S.R. Joshi, S. Sadikot, R. Gupta, S. Gulati and Y.P. Munjal. (2009) "Consensus Statement for Diagnosis of Obesity, Abdominal Obesity and the Metabolic Syndrome for Asian Indians and Recommendations for

Physical Activity, Medical and Surgical Management". *J Assoc Physicians India*, Feb., Concensus Group, 57: 163–70.

Nambiar, V., Chauhan, S. and Daniel, M. (2010). Polyphends from Dark Chocolates and their Effects and the Nutritional Status of the Middle Aged Gujarati Jains. *International Journal of Pharmaceutical and Biological Archives* 1(2): 1–8.

Nambiar, V.S. and Guin, P. (2007) "Prevalence of Hyperglycemia and Hyperlipidemia among the Middle Aged and Elderly Population in a University Setup". *Indian J Geron*., 21 (1), pp. 30–43.

Nambiar, V.S., Mehta R. and Daniel, M. (2005) "Polyphenol Content of Three Indian Green Leafy Vegetables". *Journal of Food Science and Technology*, Vol. 42 (6), pp. 312–315.

Nambiar, V.S. and Seshadri, S. (2004). "Dietary Patterns and its Relation to Relation to Disease Profile in Postmenopausal Women". (Part II), *Indian Journal of Gerontology*, Vol. 18 (8): 73–84.

——. (2002) "Relationship between Socio-demographic Indicators, Income, Lifestyle and Caloric Intake in Postmenopausal Women". *Indian Journal of Gerontology*, Vol. 16, Nos. 3 and 4.

Narasinga Rao, B.S. (2003) "Bioactive Phytochemicals in Indian Foods and their Potential in Health Promotion and Disease Prevention". *Asia Pacific J Clinical Nutrition*, Vol. 12 (1): 9–22.

Patel, V. and Seshadri, S. (1992) Nutritional Status of Women Aged 45–58 yr from Affluent and Middle Income Groups in an Urban Setting in India. Unpublished M.Sc (Nutrition) Dissertation, Department of Foods and Nutrition. M.S. University of Baroda, Vadodara.

Seshadri, S. and Nambiar, V.S. (2003) "Kanjero (*Digera arvensis*) and Drumstick Leaves (*Moringa oleifera*): Nutrient Profile and Potential for Human Consumption", in Karger Basel (ed.), "Plants in Human Health and Nutrition Policy". *World Review of Nutrition and Dietetics*, Vol. 91: 41–56.

Strain, J.J. and I.I.F. Benjic. (1999) "Diet and Antioxidant Defence", in M.O. Sedler (ed.), *Encyclopedia of Human Nutrition*. Vol. I, New York: Academic Press, pp. 95–105.

http://www.lifehack.org/articles/lifestyle/top-ten-rejuvenating-and-anti-ageing-foods.html

18

Time-Use Pattern of Women in the Third Age

MANEESHA SHUKUL AND VEENA GANDOTRA

'Third age'—more commonly understood as old age—is termed so considering 'childhood' as the 'first age', and 'adulthood' as the 'second age'. Those above the age of 60 years are commonly considered as elderly or people in the 'third age'. The proportion of the people has increased throughout the 20th century. It has been estimated that the elderly population of the world would increase to 112.96 million by the year 2016 (Das and Shah, 2001). An estimate states that in the first 20 years of the 21st century, the number of people aged over 60 and above is expected to increase to over 1,000 million (Bond and Coleman, 1993). This increase is most likely to occur in India and China, due to the already large population base (Das and Shah, 2001). This trend started early in the industrialized nations like the US and the UK but the developing nations were also witnessing the same change. This demographic transition was a result of the decreasing mortality rates along with lengthening life expectancy, due to medical advancement. The gender differential in life expectancy has widened over the years. The female population shows a greater increase in the expected life span in all age groups as compared to the male population. The United Nations projects that by the year 2025 there will be 604 million women over the age of 60 in the world population. Seventy per cent of these will be in the Third World countries. It becomes necessary to differentiate between old men and women as gender is a powerful factor affecting the quality of life at all the stages of life. The gender, social status and martial status determine the quality of life in later years.

Women in the developing world experience low social status, poor reproductive health care, economic dependence, malnutrition and domestic violence which affect their well-being adversely. Elderly women in India are highly vulnerable due to decreasing physical capacity and mobility, increasing financial and psychological dependence, lack of availability of support network and ignorance about their rights.

Traditionally, in the Indian culture old age generally refers to being detached from the occupation, property or role in the society and family responsibilities, handing over to younger generation, occupying oneself in the realm of God. The third age is characterized by the period of retirement from the active gainfully employed life and/or hectic household work. The women's work and time-use pattern generally change in the third age. If they were employed gainfully outside the home, their time and activity pattern changes as soon as they retire. Even with the arrival of daughter-in-law in the house, the time and activity pattern generally changes, she takes part or full load of the household work. But if the daughter-in-law is gainfully employed, the work and time pattern of women in the third age may be moulded in different pattern. If the elder women have daughters only, who leave the house after marriage, then they may have to take all the workload on their own shoulder, which, otherwise was shared by their daughters. In any case, the time-use pattern undergoes changes than what was there in the earlier life.

The changing pattern raises problems of adjustment. The women in third age may need guidance to make the transition easy.

It becomes essential to find out the change in the time use pattern of women in the third age, the problems they face and be given guidance, if needed. With this background a study was undertaken with the following objectives.

Objectives of the Study

1. To study demographic characteristics of the women in the third age living in Vadodara city.
2. To study the time-use pattern of women in the third age.

3. To find out the reasons for their employment in the present life.
4. To find out monetary contribution of women in the third age through household work.

Methodology

The present study was a descriptive survey; conducted in Vadodara city having population of more than 13 lakh, of which 6.19 per cent make up people above 60 years of age with almost an equal number of males and females. Through stratified sampling 180 women in the third age were selected as sample from the list obtained through a few senior citizens' clubs/associations and old women identified through snowball technique. The old women were divided into two age groups: (i) young-old with the age range of 60–75 years, and (ii) old-old group having age of 75 years and above. Among these 30 were living alone, 30 with spouse and 30 living with family from each of the age groups.

The data were collected in the year 2003 through an interview schedule which contained questions to elicite background in formation, and questions related to time-use pattern. The data were analysed using descriptive and relational statistics.

Major Findings

Background information: Information about age, education, martial status etc. of the women in the third age is reported here.

Age: Half of the respondents were between 60 and 74 years rest between 75 years old. It was found that among the young-old respondents (between the age group of 60 to 75 years) more were in the age group of 60 to 64 years as compared to other categories (Table 1). Amongst old-old more were in the age group of 75 to 80 years.

Education: Very few respondents were illiterate. More than one third were primary pass and one-fifth were graduates.

Marital status: Half of the respondents were married, i.e., their husbands were present. Many were widowed.

Type of family: Majority were living in nuclear family.

Occupation at present: A wide majority of the respondents were not working at present. Those who were working they were doing some home-based business for about 5 to 6 hours per day. Many

Table 1 *Frequency and Percentage Distribution of Respondents as per their Background Information*

	Characteristics	Respondents (n=180)	
		f	%
A	Age		
	Young-Old		
	60–64	40	22.2
	65–69	24	13.3
	70–74	26	14.4
	Old-Old		
	75–80	56	31.2
	81–84	22	12.2
	> 85	12	6.7
B	Education		
	Illiterate	5	2.7
	Primary	65	3.6
	10th Pass	28	15.6
	12th Pass	12	6.7
	Graduate	38	21.1
	Post-Graduate	32	17.8
C	Marital Status		
(i)	Unmarried	9	5.0
(ii)	Married	92	51.1
(iii)	Widowed	77	42.8
(iv)	Divorced/Separated	2	1.1
D	Type of Family		
	Nuclear	124	69.1
	Joint	54	30.1
	N.A. (No family members living)	2	1.1
E	Occupation		
	working at present	25	13.9
	Not working	155	86.12

respondents were doing voluntary activities for 3 to 4 hours (n=33, i.e., 36.7%) from total sample.

The respondents were asked to opine whether it is necessary for older people to work (Table 2). More respondents were not able to clearly answer. They were of the opinion that older people should work if they are able to. About 16 per cent said that they should not work, there is no need/they should rest. About one-tenth of the respondents said that older people should work as they can keep their mind active. A few said that it is necessary for older people to work as they can make productive use of time.

Table 2 *Opinion about Necessity for Older People to Work*

Necessity to Work	*Comment*	*Young-Old n=90*		*Old-Old n=90*		*Total n=180*	
		f	*%*	*f*	*%*	*f*	*%*
Yes	It keeps mind active	13	14.4	4	4.4	8	9.4
	It keeps productive use of time	7	7.8	6	6.7	6	7.2
	It makes person self-reliant	1	1.1	2	2.2	1	1.1
No	No need/should rest	15	16.7	13	14.4	14	15.5
	Cannot work because of age	13	14.4	18	20.0	16	17.7
	Should leave attachment of world	2	2.2	2	2.2	2	2.2
Undecided	should work. If able to work	39	43.3	41	45.6	40	44.4
	Depends on financial status	8	8.9	6	6.7	7	7.8
	Not required for all	3	3.3	1	1.1	2	2.2

Majority of the respondents were not working in their second age, i.e., before 60 years.

Among those who were working were from the young-old age group (Table 3).

Table 3 *Information about Employment in Earlier Age*

Employment in Early Age	*Young-Old n=90*		*Old-Old n=90*		*Total n=180*	
	f	*%*	*f*	*%*	*f*	*%*
Working	44	48.9	20	22.2	32	35.5
Not Working	46	51.1	70	77.8	58	64.4

Time-Use Pattern

The women's work and time-use pattern generally change in the third age. If they were employed gainfully outside the home, their time and activity pattern changes as soon as they retire. Even with the arrival of daughter-in-law in the house or the daughters leaving the house after marriage or for studies, the time and activity pattern generally changes. However, in case she is gainfully employed, the work and time pattern of women in third age may be moulded in different pattern. It is essential to study whether there is any change in the time and activity pattern of women in the third age, so that, if needed, guidance can be given to overcome the problems they face.

Table 4 *Change in the Time-Use Pattern*

Change in the Time-Use Pattern		*Living Arrangement*									
		Living Alone n=60		*Living with Husband n=60*		*Living with Family n=60*		*Total*		*Total Sample n=180*	
		f	%	*f*	%	*f*	%	*f*	%	*f*	%
Young-Old	Changed	27	90.0	23	76.7	23	76.7	73	81.1	152	84.4
	Not Changed	3	10.0	7	23.3	7	23.3	17	18.9	28	15.6
	Total	30	100.0	30	100.0	30	100.0	90	100.00		
Old-Old	Changed	27	90.0	27	90.0	25	83.3	79	87.8		
	Not Changed	3	10.0	3	10.0	5	16.7	11	12.2		
	Total	30	100.0	30	100.0	30	100.0	90	100.0		

Almost 85 per cent of the elderly women across the young and old age groups felt that their time-use pattern had changed after attaining 60 years of age (Table 4). A wide majority of the women whether they lived alone or were living with husband or family, said that their time and activity pattern has changed.

Reasons for Change in Time-Use Pattern

The respondents were asked the reasons for changing their time and activity pattern after the age of 60 years. About 43 per cent of women felt that the change in time and activity pattern was due to health-related conditions. There were more old-old women than young-old women who gave this reason (Table 5). One-fourth of women felt the change due to retirement.

Table 5 *Reasons for Change in Time-Use Pattern*

Reasons for Change in Time-Use Pattern	*Young-Old n=90*		*Old-old n=90=100*		*Total n=180*	
	f	*%*	*f*	*%*	*f*	*%*
Retirement	28	31.3	17	18.9	45	25.0
Arrival of daughter-in-law	16	17.8	24	26.7	40	22.2
Health	26	28.9	51	56.7	77	42.8
Death of spouse	8	8.9	7	7.8	15	8.3
Dependency on children	3	10.0	0	0	3	1.66
Marriage of daughter	5	5.6	0	0	5	2.8
Retirement of spouse	1	3.3	3	10.0	4	2.2
Family problems	4	4.4	0	0	4	2.2

Table 6 *Time Spent on Various Activities Before and After 60 Years of Age by Young-Old Women*

	Young-Old Women (60 to 75 Years)							
Activities	*Time Spent Per Day in hours Before*				*Time Spent Per Day in hours After*			
	LA	*LH*	*LF*	*Total*	*LA*	*LH*	*LF*	*Total*
Work	6.73	7.55	6.12	6.8	4.17	2.63	2.17	2.99
Household work	4.16	4.69	3.82	4.22	3.62	4.21	2.76	3.53
Leisure/recreation	2.55	2.27	1.76	2.19	2.78	3.15	2.45	2.79
Personal care	0.82	0.76	0.66	0.73	1.13	1.16	0.76	1.02
Eating	0.62	0.72	0.85	0.73	0.69	0.83	0.91	0.81
Social activities	2.47	1.97	1.71	2.05	2.46	1.91	1.73	2.03
Rest/sleep	5.27	6.58	4.5	5.45	5.22	7.1	4.96	5.76
Religious activities	1.37	0.99	1.06	1.13	1.58	1.28	2.08	1.65
Family interaction	2.35	2.92	1.91	2.39	1.90	3.92	2.20	2.67

(Key: LA=Living alone; LH = Living with Husband; LF = Living with Family)

There were little less than one-fourth of the respondents who said that with the arrival of daughter-in-law the change was felt. This was reported by more of old-old women than the young-old women.

Time and Activities Pattern: Before and After

An enquiry was made as to how much time the women spent on various activities per day. The responses were subjective and based on the recall method.

Among the young-old respondents time spent work decreased after 60 years of age (Table 6). There was a slight decrease in the time spent for household work. On the other hand, there was some increase in the time spent for leisure/recreation. Especially among those who lived with their husbands and families. Their time for family interactions also increased. The time spent on personal care also increased after 60 years of age amongst all the women irrespective of their living condition.

Table 7 *Time Spent on Various Activities Before and After 60 years of Age by Old-Old Women*

Activities	*Old-Old Women (60 to 75 Years)*							
	Time Spent Per Day in hours Before 60 Years				*Time Spent Per Day in hours After 60 Years*			
	LA	*LH*	*LF*	*Total*	*LA*	*LH*	*LF*	*Total*
Work	7.58	7.17	8.2	7.65	3.5	5.75	4.5	3.08
Household work	3.44	3.80	4.23	3.82	1.97	2.19	1.95	2.03
Leisure/Recreation	1.91	1.92	2.2	2.01	3.61	2.65	2.98	3.08
Personal care	0.89	0.87	1.16	0.97	0.87	0.94	0.63	0.81
Eating	0.56	0.71	0.45	0.57	0.60	0.71	0.47	0.59
Social Activities	1.94	2.61	2.5	2.35	2.0	2.68	1.80	2.16
Rest/Sleep	5.08	4.52	3.86	4.48	5.65	5.09	4.82	5.19
Religious Activities	1.44	1.07	1.44	1.32	1.80	1.52	1.65	1.66
Family Interaction	1.91	2.14	2.02	2.02	2.02	2.65	2.92	2.51

(Key: LA=Living alone; LH = Living with Husband; LF = Living with Family).

Time spent for work and household work decreased and leisure time/recreation increased (Table 7). Slightly it increased for religious activities. Not much change in time-use pattern was reported by women having 75 years and above age.

Thus, it was observed that the time spent on work and household work decreased but that on leisure/recreation, family interaction increased and slight increase in the rest/sleep. This may be because of retirement from gainful employment and arrival of a helping hand, that of a daughter-in-law in the house. About 22 per cent respondents gave this reason for change in the time-use pattern, (see Table 5). Another reason can be the problems of deteriorating health which might have reduced their activities (43% respondents gave this reason, see Table 5).

Monetary Contribution of Women in the Third Age through Household Work

To find out how much monetary contribution old or women make to the family, the market-value was applied to various kinds of work. For this it was assumed that for the same kind of work, if a hired help (maid servant) was employed, then, what would be the expenditure incurred by the household. This methodology is similar to one of the methodologies evolved in the estimation of national income the contribution of women through the household work. This approach, though has certain limitations, but, gives fair idea about the worth of an elderly person in the family.

For the purpose of evaluating the monetary contribution of the elderly towards the family, selected household tasks were considered based on the total percentage of time spent on activities. The findings showed that cooking (60%), cleaning of house (40%), cleaning utensils (18.3%), laundry (35%) cutting vegetables (56%) and general supervision (31.1%) being major household activities.

There were multiple responses.

Table 8 *Monetary Contribution of Elderly Women Towards Family*

Activities	*No. of Respondents*	*Cost of Hired help (per month)*	*Total Monetary Contribution*
1	*2*	*3*	*4 = 2 × 3*
Cooking	108	1,500	1,62,000
Cleaning of house	72	300	21,600
Cleaning utensils	33	250	8,250
Laundry	62	250	3,875
Cutting vegetables	101	20	2,020
General supervision	56	150	8,400
Total	432	2,470	2,06,145

The cost of hiring help was multiplied with the number of respondents. The total was found to be Rs 2,06,145. If, divided by the number of total respondents, the average comes to about 477.17, i.e., Rs 500 approximately. Thus, on an average, it can be stated that this amount they are contributing towards their household, or rather saving from the monthly expenditure made by the family.

Conclusion

The women in the third age find their time-use pattern changed from that time when they were less than 60 years old. This change was attributed to the health, retirement and arrival of daughter-in-law in the home. The time spent on work and household work decreased remarkably from before to after the age of 60 years. Their time on leisure, family interaction, and religious activities increased. Those elderly women who have good health should be motivated and facilitated to do more productive work, may be voluntary, for the society.

References

Bond, John and Peter Coleman. (1999) *Ageing in Society: An Introduction to Social Gerontology*. Sage Publications, London.

Das, N.P. and U. Shah. (2001) "The Social and Mental Status of the Elderly in India: Evidence from Recent National Level Data". *PRC*, December.

19

Safety Measures for Elderly in Old Age Homes

SHEWANTI N. KASHYAP

The Indian population has increased from 361 million in 1951 to 1.027 billion in 2001. Simultaneously, the number of older people has increased from 19 million (4% of total population) to 77 million (7.5% of the total) during the same time span (Registrar General of India). India, like many traditional societies, today faces a unique situation in providing care for its elderly as the existing old-age support structures in the form of family, kith and kin, are fast eroding and the elderly are ill-equipped to cope alone with their lives in the face of infirmity and disability. The onus of caring for the elderly is therefore now much more on the state than the family and will necessitate the creation of adequate institutional support. Elderly people living independently without any assistance and palliative measures should be considered for improving the safety within their homes, as elderly people are more prone to serious injuries and long-term disability if they fall. There is, therefore, an urgent need to examine the various aspects of this new and fast growing population to ensure the design of appropriate policy and programmes directed to meet the varied needs of this vulnerable and dependent group. In order to study the implications of an ageing population in India, the changing Indian demographic configuration needs to be highlighted first. As per recent statistics, there are 1,018 old age homes in India today. Out of these, 427 homes are free of cost while 153 old age homes are on pay and stay basis, 146 homes have both free as well as pay and stay facilities and detailed information is not available for 292 homes. A total of 371 old age homes all over the country are available for the sick and 118 homes are exclusive for women. A majority of the old age homes are concentrated in the developed states including Gujarat (Directory of Old Age Homes in India, Help India, 2002). It has been found out that many old age homes were not conducive to the old because of unsuitable landscape and surroundings. These homes were also lacking in basic and support facilities. Apart from these, this group also has the right to live with society enabling them to lead normal lives in a safe and comfortable environment. The design of the structural environment should support, rather than restrict, a person's daily life. It also allows for the individual to meet physical, psychological and social needs, and promote a sense of well-being and safety. As an older person requires attentive care and special treatment, there is an urgent need to provide a comfortable living to elderly through old age homes by simple modification in designing the old age homes and carefully selecting the infrastructural facilities, the recommendations are as under:

Fittings and Fixtures

Installation of door level handles, larger and well located electric switches, visual as well as auditory alarm system, sliding doors (particularly for cabinet and cupboard), pull-push handles, and handrails along both sides of building corridors are essential requirements in old age homes.

Bath Fixtures

- A raised toilet seat with hand grips on both sides helps. Also, showers should be of non-slip material underfoot and grips at both standing and sitting level.
- The toilet should be positioned next to a sidewall to allow the installation of an assist grab bar.
- Provide a toilet with a seat height of about 18 inches (the standard is 16 inches).
- Avoid the available high seat toilets that are 20"; the feet of a short person may not reach the floor.

- The electric vent fan either wall or ceiling mounted, gravity flow vents, and shafts that allow air to escape to the outside.

Toilet

The standard 15 to 17 inch height of toilet seats creates a problem for many people, especially those with arthritis, hip, knee or back problems. Elevating the seat from 5 to 7 inches will give better leverage in regaining a standing position. There are several types of removable and permanently fixed raised toilet seats available. Two examples are:

- A molded plastic seat (see Figure 1) is the simplest way to increase seat height by about 4 inches
- An adjustable seat (see Figure 2) will add from 3 to 6 inches of height.
- For a more permanent raised toilet, a plumber can put the stool on a wooden platform made to fit the toilet bowl base (see Figure 3).

  If building a new bathroom, consider a wall-hung toilet (see Figure 4) that can be hung at any height.

Special Feature (Portable Bidets)

Figure 1 *Molded Plastic Seat*

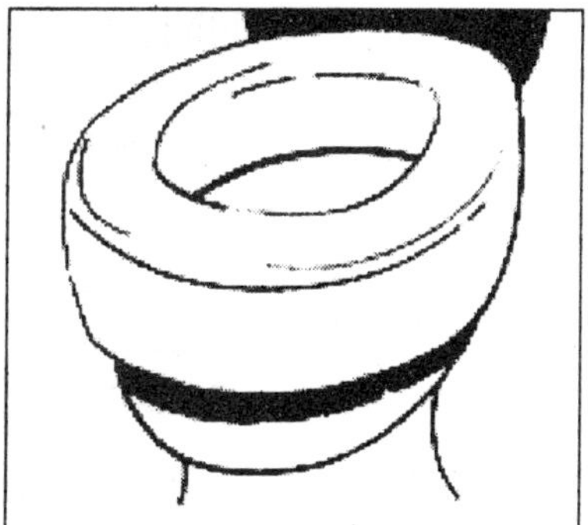

Figure 2 *Adjustable Seats*

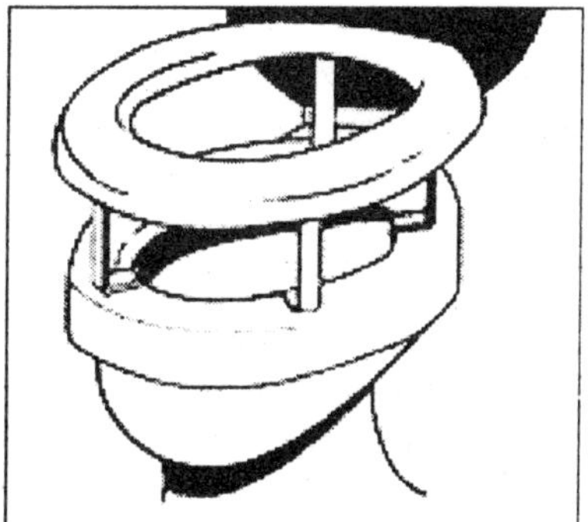

A special unit (portable bidet) for cleaning the perinea area without hands or paper may be attached to any standard toilet bowl (see Figure 5). It is an electrically powered unit with a mechanism for spray washing with warm water and drying with a flow of warm air.

Figure 3 *Raised Toilet Base*

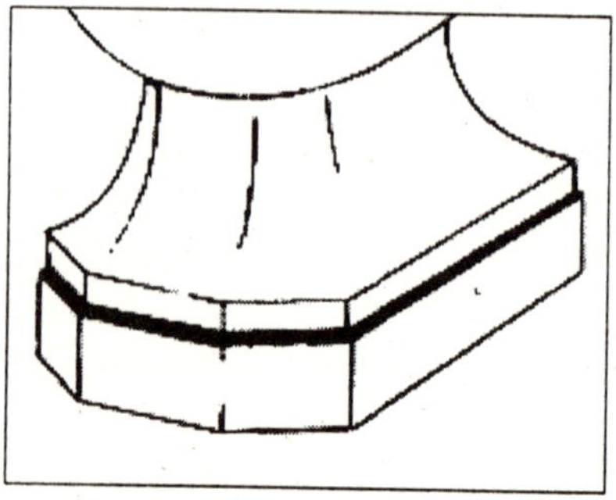

Figure 4 *Wall Hung Toilet*

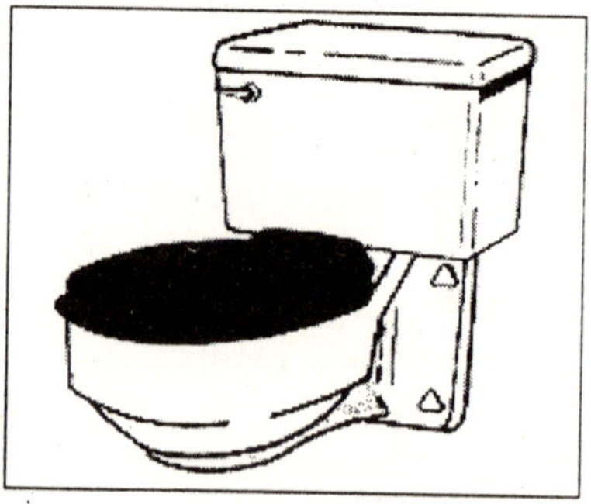

This promotes independence for persons with very limited hand/arm functions.

Figure 5 *Portable Bidets*

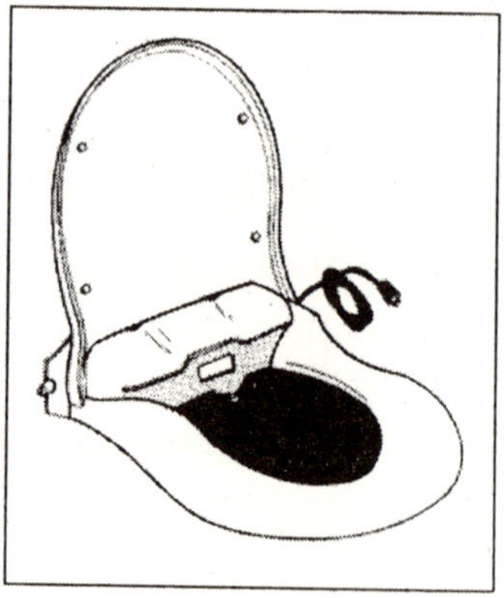

Grab Bars

Grab bars around the toilets are for safety. Many types are available. The choice will depend on: (1) available wall space near the toilet; (2) nearness to other fixtures in the room; and (3) needs of people in the household. Basic types of toilet support bars include:

- Wall-mounted on the back wall behind the toilet (see Figure 6).
- Wall/floor mounted (see Figure 7).
- Slipover guard rails (see Figure 10).
- Other safety features.

Lighting Fixtures

Good lighting not only assists with reading and safety, it helps prevent depression for those confined indoors.

- A flashlight at bedside and night lights along the route to the bathroom are essential and pay for themselves in accidents prevented.
- If cost is a concern, the improved, inexpensive fluorescent light bulbs may be satisfactory.

Figure 6 *Side and back Mounted Bars*

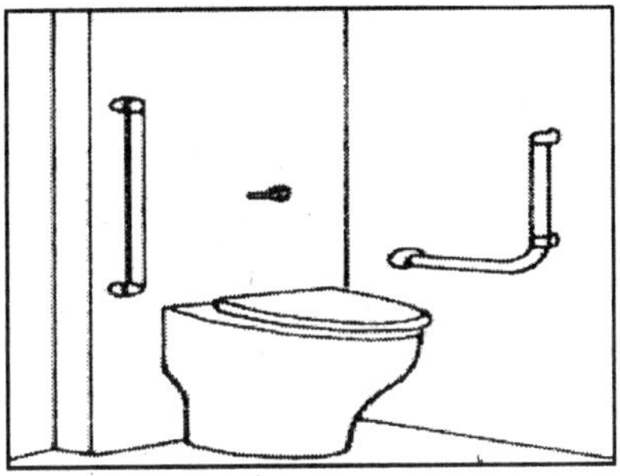

Figure 7 *Wall/Floor Mounted*

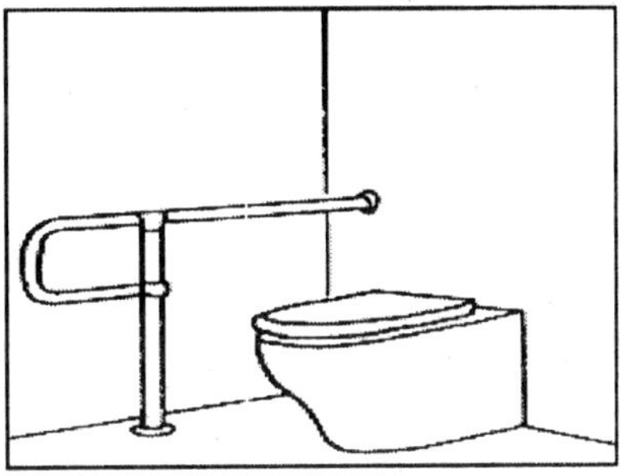

Figure 8 *Free Standing*

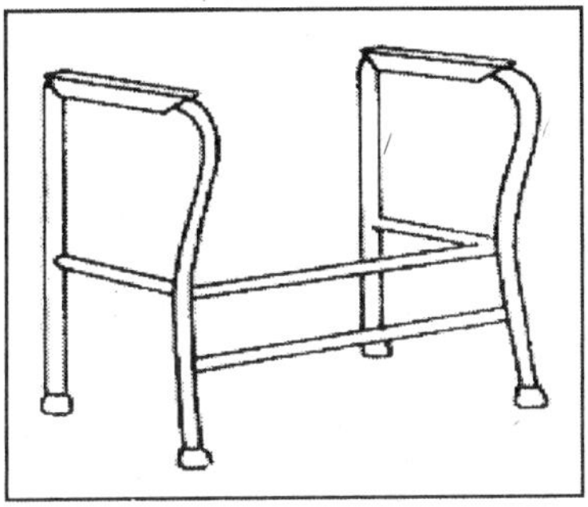

Figure 9 *Floor Model*

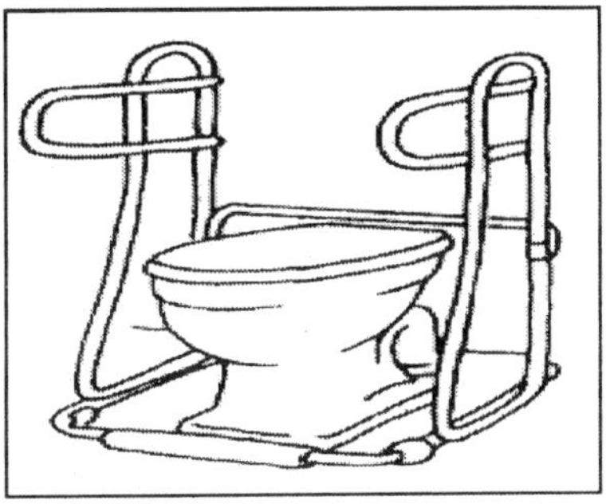

Figure 10 *Slipovers*

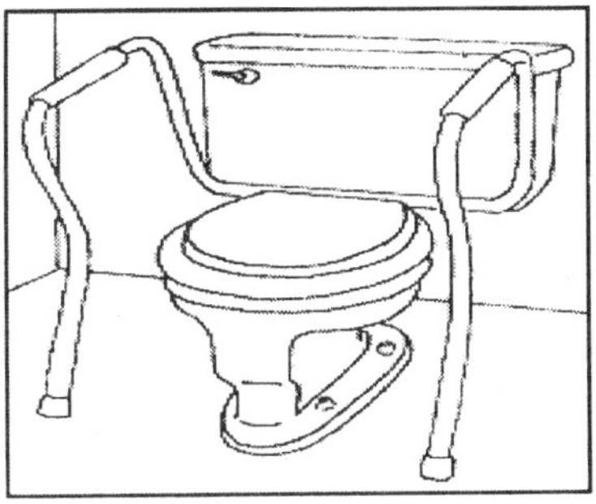

Figure 11 *Single Lever Faucets*

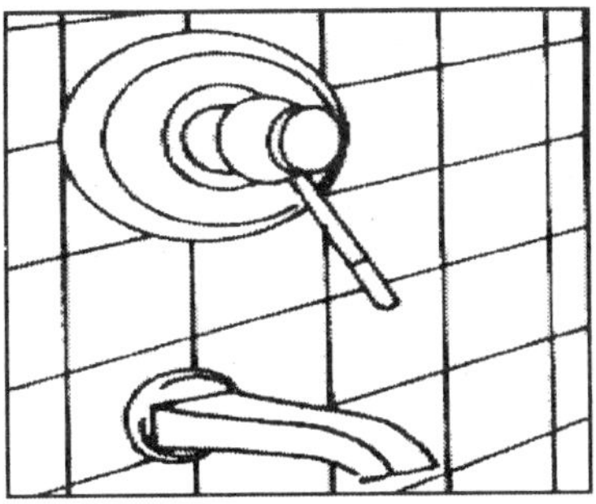

- The stairs should be well illuminated by natural or artificial light. A light switch should be located at each end of the stairs. The fixtures should not cause glare, nor should it cause any shadows.
- Wall fixtures are preferred over ceiling fixtures for easier and safer bulb changing. Provide night lights in hallways and bathrooms.

Environmental Safety

It can be maximized through sound insulation; improvement in residential temperature control would avert temperature extremes. Maintain a relative humidity of 30–70 per cent at 65–75 degrees Fahrenheit to accommodate a decrease in thermal range tolerance that comes with age.

Furniture and Furnishing

The types of furniture chosen for a facility can impact on a person's mobility and, therefore, their independence. Furniture is also a safety concern for the elderly because older people are often prone to falls due to general weakening as a person ages.

Here are some points to keep in mind regarding furniture in a facility:

- Special care should be taken in selection of furniture and furnishing at old age homes.
- The chair redesigning can be done with proper cushioning and back rest with slop of 110°–115° angles with arm and foot rest.
- Lightweight chairs with high arms will help a person move the chair while seated in it.
- The arms of chairs need to extend to the edge of the seat to facilitate pushing off. Chair arms should have flat tops and ends designed for grasping.
- A high back on a chair will decrease the chance of falling backward for those people who rock to get out of a chair.
- A seating height of 17–18 inches and a seating depth of 18–19 inches will allow a person's feet to touch the ground without putting pressure behind their knees.
- The bottoms of chairs should be open so a person's feet can be tucked underneath as their weight is shifted forward to stand.
- Chairs with casters are unsafe and should not be used.

- A redesign of current operating room tables may be required to meet the ergonomic guidelines, table height should be 66.6 cm.
- A round table with a sturdy pedestal base will allow more seating space with the ability to adjust for wheelchairs.
- The bed should not be too low/high, it can be an appropriate height for easy transfer on and off. The metal cots can be replaced with wooden with thick mattresses to avoid back pain.
- Beds should be set-up so that when seated at the side of the bed, a person's feet will rest firmly on the floor with their legs at right angles.
- Mattresses should have firm edges to make getting in and out of bed easier and decrease the occurrences of falls.
- Use an attachable handrail on beds when needed. The handrail should attach securely to the frame, be height-adjustable, and swivel and lock in place.
- Consider alternatives to standard spring and coil mattresses, such as an "opencell" foam mattress or a large-celled alternating pressure mattress, in facilities where pressure ulcers may be a concern. Sheepskin pads or rubberized sheets with a soft backing can also be used.
- The wooden walking cane should be with a crook handle and length adjustable from 74 cm to 97 cm.
- Furnishings should be stable, with rounded corners for safety.
- A variety of heights should be available for counters and shelves.

To help ensure that Home Sweet Home is also Home Safe Home, the following ABCs for safe home furnishings should be followed:

- A is for awareness, which can help prevent accidents in the home.
- B is for bunk beds, a good choice for children aged 6 and older.
- C is for cribs, the best place for your baby to sleep. Make sure slats or spindles are no more than 2.4 inches apart and that none are loose or missing. The mattress should be firm and fit snugly in the crib.
- D is for drawers, great for stashing your stuff, but terrible as a stepping stool. To prevent tip over, never allow children to climb in drawers or open more than one at a time. Automatic drawer stops, which keep drawers from falling out on unsuspecting feet, are often a good feature, especially if children are in the home.

- E is for entertainment centre, the perfect place to house your new TV. Just be sure it is the right size so that the TV is properly supported and would not fall forward.
- F is for falls, a leading cause of injuries and deaths in the home. Particularly vulnerable are the elderly. To lessen the likelihood of falls, eliminate clutter, be sure rugs have slip-resistant pads, keep electrical cords out of walkways and clean up spills immediately.
- G is for guardrails. Bunk beds should have guardrails on each side of the top bunk, with the side against the wall or opposite the ladder running the full length of the bed. The other rail should have no more than 15 inches open at each end. Rails should be secure and sturdy and should extend at least 5 inches above the top of the mattress.
- H is for height, which you should consider in bookcases and dressers. If the piece is taller than it is wide, you may want to secure it to the wall to prevent tip over, especially if young children are in the home. And bookcases should never be overloaded, particularly on top.
- I is for ideal. Remember that the ideal furnishings for your home are not only comfortable and beautiful, but safe as well.
- J is for joiners. It is a good idea to check periodically to make sure all screws, bolts, brackets and other joiners on your furniture are tight and secure.
- K is for kids, who love to play but who should never be allowed to play or climb on furniture, especially on bunk beds, dressers or open reclining chairs.
- L is for lids and latches. Toy and storage chests should have safety latches that prevent the lid from falling freely or slamming shut on fingers or a child's head. Lids should not lock automatically. If you have an older chest without a safety latch, contact the manufacturer for a replacement latch, or remove the lid.
- M is for matches. Careless smoking is the third leading cause of fires.
- N is for night time, when it gets dark. When the sun goes down, lighting should come on. Use a variety of floor and table lamps, as well as ceiling and wall fixtures, to ensure that your home is well-lit so people can move around safely. Candles are a nice touch for evening, but use caution near upholstery and bedding.

- O is for old, which could be dangerous. Be sure older pieces of furniture do not contain lead paint that is flaking. Also check for sturdiness and stability.
- P is for pathways, which should be clutter free and well-lit, both inside and outside the home. Furniture should be arranged to allow easy walk through.
- Q is for quality. Buy the best you can afford—for safety's sake. Quality furniture, regardless of price range, is manufactured with safety in mind.
- R is for recliner, a comfortable seat, but one that requires caution. Only one adult should sit in a recliner at a time, and children should never be allowed to play on or around a recliner. To prevent cuts and lacerations, do not put your hands or fingers under the mechanism to operate the chair.
- S is for supervision, for which there is no substitute. No matter how safe the products in your home are, small children should always be supervised by a responsible adult.
- T is for temptation, which should be avoided. To prevent tempting your children to climb on furniture, do not place enticing objects on tops of dressers or bookcases.
- U is for UFAC, the Upholstered Furniture Action Council. When buying new upholstered furniture, look for the gold UFAC tag ensuring that the manufacturer has agreed to meet UFAC's construction criteria. The voluntary UFAC programme has been credited with contributing to a nearly 80 per cent reduction in the number of upholstered furniture fires started by smoldering cigarettes.
- V is for vigilant, which is what you should be when it comes to home safety.
- W is for windows, which provide a wonderful view. But furniture, especially children's beds, should not be placed near windows where children can climb or fall out.
- X is for X-ing out accidents in your home. Following these simple ABC tips will lead you on your way to safety at home.
- Y is for yawning, leading us to ...
- Z, which is for the great ZZZs you will catch when you know your are safe at home.

Colour Codes

There was lack of colour codes and visual contrast and this can be achieved either through brightness or colour difference to make the key features more perceptible.

- Paint doors and their trim a contrasting colour from the walls. Door thresholds should be flush with the floor, or painted a contrasting colour. Doors left halfway open can be dangerous. One way to solve this problem is with gentle self-closing devices.
- Interior colour schemes with good contrast help elderly people with diminishing eye sight identify doors, entrance ways and changed surface conditions.
- Switch plates, and electrical sockets, that are of contrasting colour from the wall will be easier to see. Use light shades of paint on walls. Flat finishes help eliminate glare.
- Light filtering curtains, blinds, shades and awnings cut down on glare through windows, but allow plenty of indirect sunlight into the house.
- Safety architectural symbols should be marked for electric installation like fuse board, fan, regulator, switch outlets and so forth.

Design Requirements

Home modifications are adaptations to one's living environment that are intended to increase the client's ease of using the home and encourage feelings of safety, security and independence. The objective of home modification is to accommodate those with decreased capacity due to a decline in health, by reducing the demands that the physical environment exerts on their daily activities. Home modifications can include changes or additions to the structural layout of the home, such as widening doorways; installing special equipment like grab bars, handrails and ramps; changing the layout of furniture; and adjusting the way the clients use their homes, such as moving to the bedroom to the first floor or changing the use of a room. Elimination of level differences, rounded corners and edges, easily operable facilities like accessible storage spaces (cabinet, cupboard and rack).

Stairs and Steps

Stairs and steps both indoors and out are formidable obstacles to many elderly people and are the location of many seriously debilitating accidents. Stairs and steps should be avoided in environments designed for the elderly people or minimized as much as possible and these can be replaced by providing stair lift.

- Handrails should be placed on both sides of the stairs, even within the dwelling unit.
- The rail should extend beyond the steps at the top and the bottom

Design consideration should be more for female than male as the female survive and suffer more. Knowledge about the biomechanical, physiological, and psychological effects of ageing is needed when designing ergonomic spaces for the elderly. A regular visit to old age homes by geriatric doctors and nursing care such as dressing, medication and injection, etc., are highly needed. The old age homes cannot offer the same satisfaction as the person's own home, but the institutional environment can be enhanced through the following:

- An attractive décor.
- Inclusion of the individual's personal possessions.
- Respect for privacy and personal territory.
- Recognition of the individuality of the resident.
- Allowance of maximum control over activities and decision-making.
- Environmental modifications to compensate for deficits.
- Social, recreational and educational activities provided to develop their potential to promote a family atmosphere and to enhance mutual support among elderly people.

As we reach our later years we can start to feel more vulnerable within our homes. Often, this is simply due to us being less mobile and more at risk of suffering a fall slip or trip but there are other factors which elderly people and their families should also consider.

Falls, Slips and Trips

Accidents in the home unfortunately tend to occur more frequently and become more distressing as we get older. Falls, slips and trips are the most common cause of physical injury to the elderly but the risks of them occurring can be reduced if we take some precautionary measures. Handrails in all the key locations such as the stairs, front and back doors and the bath and toilet can make keeping your balance much easier and you should also ensure that any rugs you use in these kinds of areas have non-slip mats underneath them. Better still, if you can live without a rug, that is even better as, even with slip mats, the corners of a rug can become worn and turn upwards over time which is a potential trip hazard. Keep all of the rooms well lit. In dimly lit rooms, it may be difficult to see any hazards so you should use bulbs which are 100W. Low energy light bulbs might seem expensive but they will last far longer than conventional light bulbs and the additional expense is worth it. Keeping a generally tidy and orderly home is also important. This does not necessarily mean vacuuming and polishing every day but simple things like keeping any wires that you could trip over hidden away and keeping a storage area, perhaps a spare room, in which you can store all of your clutter. Not only will you find things more easily if they are all in the same place, it will stop you are tripping over them. Moping up all spills immediately will also reduce the chances of slipping. You should also remove any casters from furniture where possible. This will make furniture more stable for you to hold onto for balance or to lean against. And, always seek help if you are uncertain about taking on a particular chore in the house. For example, putting up curtains or changing light bulbs. Providing you are not disabled, you should try to keep as active as possible as regular exercise improves balance, coordination and strength.

Waterproof Walls and Floors

The type of material you select for your walls and floors can make a difference. Obviously, the countertop and walls should be waterproof and easy to clean. Flooring should be heavy duty to cater for heavy traffic and be water-resistant. Ceramic tiles are a common choice as they are excellent water buffers. You can create striking patterns on the walls through the use of tiles. You do not have to tile your whole bathroom, although it does make it easier to clean. You can instead tile the bottom half of the wall and use paint for the top half. Washable semi-gloss enamel type paint is best. High gloss paints, although easier to wash and clean, may be too overpowering for a small bathroom.

The floor surface contributes too many trips and falls.

- Extra power points eliminate the tangle of loose extension leads that can cause unexpected falls.

- Eliminate unnecessary changes in floor levels wherever possible.
- Using more impact-absorbent floor surfaces reduces the potential level of injury caused by a fall.
- Mosaic tiles are also popular but should be used on walls instead of floors as they are slippery. Changes in floor levels must be avoided.
- Smooth floor surfaces should be minimized. In potentially wet areas such as kitchens, baths, entries or laundries, unglazed "Skid Resistance Polycemtiles" which was developed by Central Building Research Institute, Roorkee, (India), and this tile is recommended for the old age homes. The specifications are as under:

Polycemtiles

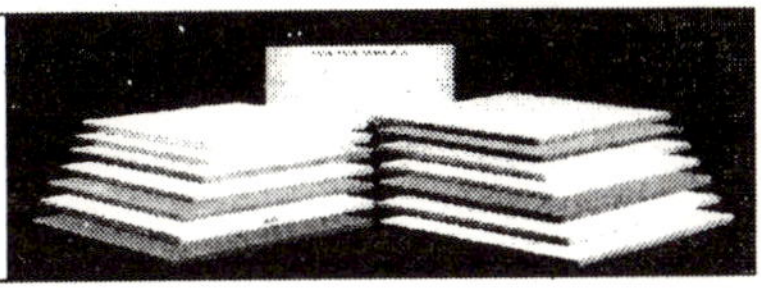

Application/uses: Suitable for floor and walls of residential, commercial and industrial buildings.

Salient technical features: Polycem tiles are prepared by combining the cement with the polymers along with some additives for biding the aggregate. There is appreciable improvement especially in physico-mechanical properties like high mechanical and wear strength, low porosity, dimensionally stable, aesthetically appealing and durable.

Environmental aspects: No adverse effect on the environment.

Level/scale of development: Laboratory scale.

Status of commercialization: Ready for commercialization.

Major components/: Raw materials Polymeric systems compatible with portland cement, siliceous and calcareous aggregate.

Major plant equipment and machinery: Mixer, blender, hydraulic press, moulds, polishing equipment.

Techno-economics: Rs 10–20 per sq ft depending upon texture and colour

Technology package: Complete design and construction know-how

Keeping Warm

Elderly people are often most at risk of suffering from illness due to cold weather and many pensioners struggle to keep up with the fuel bills, particularly in the winter. Ways of ensuring that you remain as warm as possible and to manage your fuel consumption more economically include wearing several thinner layers of clothing as opposed to one thick layer as warmth is retained better between several layers. Keeping a woolens or some other type of warm hat handy, no matter whether you feel silly or not, will also help your body to retain more heat. You should always try to have at least one hot meal per day and have regular hot drinks throughout the day. A hot drink, especially before bedtime, helps to keep your body temperature up and it is often a good idea to take a thermos flask to bed so you can have a hot drink in the night if you wake up feeling cold. Sitting ill for long periods can also make you feel cold so, if you are able, try to build some kind of exercise into your day. This is not only good for your mobility but will help you stay warm too. There are other practical things you can do to keep your home warm. Insulation, draught proofing and lagging pipes all help to stop the heat from escaping and sometimes you can get financial help from your local authority to help you with this. And, if you have central heating, it is more economical to set the time for the heating to come on a bit earlier than to push the thermostat up higher.

Security

It is a sad fact of life that burglars and intruders see frail and elderly people as 'easy targets' so it is crucial that you take security measures to reduce the risk of becoming a victim. It does not take a burglar more than a few minutes to access your property, steal valuables then leave so always lock your doors and any windows and do not be tempted to leave them unlocked just because you are 'popping next door or to the corner shop' for a few minutes. Do not be tempted to leave a spare door key in a 'hidden' place. No matter how well you think you have hidden it, burglars will always be one step ahead of you. Likewise, do not leave keys where they are clearly visible. Burglars are adept at fishing keys from a table or hook near a door or window by fishing them out using a rod and hook via your letterbox or through an open window. And, if you can clearly see into your home from the roadside, make sure that any expensive items such as computers, expensive TVs, etc., are not easily seen from outside.

Bogus Callers

Elderly people are often the target for bogus callers and many people have been duped by unscrupulous criminals claiming that they are from the council, gas workers and even from the police! Fit a chain onto your door and use it whenever somebody knocks. Ask the caller for some identification and even check that out by calling the relevant company or authority before letting them in. Do not just assume that the ID card or badge is genuine. There are some good fake ones knocking around, so call the companies up to verify the person's authenticity. If they are genuine, they would not mind waiting 5 or 10 minutes for you to make checks and even if they do mind, do not let them in without proper verification first. You may also be visited by genuine but 'hard sell' and unscrupulous sales people. Unless you are genuinely interested and have verified that they are genuine, you may end up being pressured to sign on the dotted line for something you do not really want or need and this might end up costing you thousands of rupees. A useful tip, if you might be potentially interested in what a salesperson has to offer, is not to let them in at all but ask them to give you or send you some literature so that you can make up your own mind and ask them for a number they can be contacted on so that you can come back to them, if you are genuinely interested. If they insist that it is a "once in a lifetime, here and now"' opportunity then you should kindly decline. But whether it is a salesperson or bogus caller or anyone else for that matter, use the door chain always. Remember the old adage, "if in doubt, keep them out". It could be very easy to become scared and feel even more vulnerable after reading some of this advice. However, the chances of you becoming a victim yourself are highly unlikely and these are just some extra precautionary measures to help to safeguard you further. More information can be found at organizations like Age Concern if you want to find out more.

Lawns/Gardens

Lawns should be well maintained and free of clutter. After dark pathways, stairs and entryways should be well lit. Halogen light is a good choice for outdoor lighting. Get lawn furniture that is a contrasting colour from the lawn. Use fencing to mark off steep hills or walls. Prune tree branches back to above head level. Raised bed or border gardens are easy to take care of. Garden tools with yellow or white handles are easy to find. Using mulch will keep weeds down and the garden will require less watering.

Kitchen/Laundry Room

High quality flourescent lighting is the best bet for the kitchen, laundry room, and shop. Appliances with controls on the front make life easier and safer for the visually impaired. Every thing has its place in a visually impaired persons kitchen. Moving the baking powder from one shelf to another can ruin a whole recipe. Kitchen cabinet doors left open are very dangerous. A rehabilitation teacher from an agency for the blind and visually impaired can help with adapting appliances like: stoves, microwave ovens, washers, dryers, thermostats, etc. They can also teach new cooking techniques

Shop/Utility Room

Inexpensive four-foot flourescent shop lights are a good choice for the utility room. There should be easy access to: electrical panel, furnace, hot water heater and main water shut off valves. Steam boilers, that have a glass water level indicator on them, can be adapted with an automatic refill valve. If the house has a fuse box replace it with a well-labelled circuit breaker box. If the house uses oil or propane for heating, set-up an automatic refill plan with a supplier. When building new or replacing heating systems consider using electric heat or forced hot air heat, they require no homeowner maintenance.

Clothing

Clothing that is neat and clean, fits well, and gives a feel of confidence. Older people are often concerned about their appearance. Most people like clothing that is easy to put on and take off. If a person needs help getting dressed and undressed, clothes that goes on and come off easily help everyone concerned. Many times elderly people have trouble raising their arms, bending or leaning. This makes getting dressed more painful, and is frustrating for the caregiver, as well. Clothes that fit loosely without being baggy are easier to get on and off. Features such as front openings, large zipper pulls, hook-and loop tape closures, or wrap styles may help. Clothing that is chosen with function in mind allows more comfortable movement in daily activities. While choosing the product following points should be kept in mind, the wearer's physical condition the frequency of changing required convenience of changing purchase costs time required and cost. Shoes that are too large, offer poor support, or have high heels can lead to falls, as can loose hosiery and robes or slacks that drag on the floor.

Clothing Comfort can be Classified as:

Physical comfort: Clothing protects people from humidity, heat, and cold, and helps them feel physically comfortable. Characteristics of fabric that affect physical comfort include flexibility, bulkiness, weight, and texture. Garment construction also affects physical comfort.

Psychological comfort: Clothing gives the wearer a sense of well being. It tells something about the person. Clothing also affects the way others see, think of, and react to the person.

Social comfort: A person can be comfortable or uncomfortable wearing a certain garment or type of clothing in a social situation. Social comfort may be involved when a person wishes to "make an impression" through the clothing he or she wears.

The clothing should provide comfortable of movement, ease to wear it, and easy to wash.

Recommendation for Better Clothing

- Waistlines loose enough to expand when the person is seated. If the waist is elastic, be sure it does not cut. Large neck openings.
- Accessible loose front pockets for carrying personal items.
- Use of soft cloth materials
- Winters can have loose woolen sweaters for men and women with large neck and warm head coverings.
- Loose fitting clothes are more comfortable, and are designed not to cause friction sores or bruising.
- Wider sleeves allow for greater ease of movement for men and women.
- Colours are bright and cheerful, for a better sense of health and well being.
- It should always bring dignity to the wearer, should ease the pain of dressing, and save the caregiver time and frustration.
- Use cardigans rather than pullovers, and other garments with front openings.

- Choose a spot in the room for the person to dress and a different spot for the person to get undressed and ready for bed. Try to use the same spots every day.

For Men

- Try pants with elastic waistbands.
- Tube socks are easier to put on, because they have no heels.
- T-Shirts tend to look okay even if worn backwards.
- If snaps, hooks, zippers and belt buckles are too difficult to manage, replace them with Velcro tape.
- Velcro closures on shoes allow the width to be easily adjusted for swelling.
- Cloth materials should be little stretchable as well.
- It is important to have good fitting shoes and slippers to allow safe mobility.

For Women

Try slip-on blouses, wrap-around or elastic waistband skirts or slacks. Front fastening bras are easier for you both to manage. Not wearing a bra can cause soreness and discomfort; however, a cotton vest may be considered if the person has difficulty with a bra. Older women can wear loose salwar-kameez rather than a saree, for easy dressing. In summers wear loose T shirt.

Guidelines in Occupational Safety and Health for Elderly Home Workers

Workers working at elderly homes not only take care of the meals and daily necessities of the residents, but also have to lift, hold or

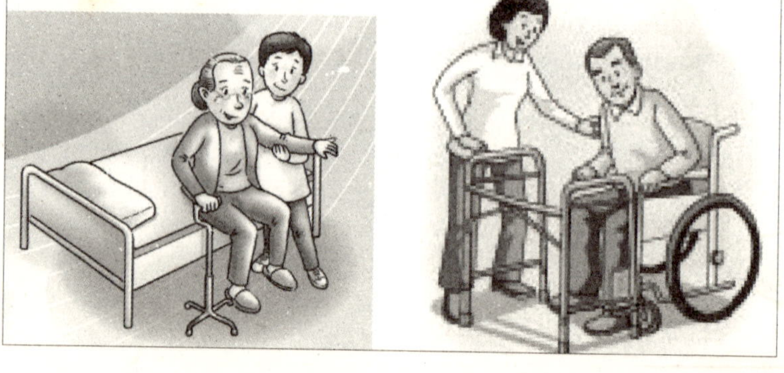

transport the elders who are infirm or incapable of mobility The Occupational Safety and Health Ordinance was enacted in May 1997 to provide for the safety and health protection of employees at work. The Occupational Safety and Health Regulation made under the Ordinance covers a wide range of basic health and safety matters as well as manual handling operations and first aid facilities. Employers are obliged to take care of the safety and health of the employees. Wherever it is reasonable and practicable, employers should eliminate the health hazards and other factors endangering the health and safety of the employees. If it is not possible to eliminate the hazards, their risks to health or safety should be reduced to the minimal. Employees should cooperate with the employers and abide by all the rules and codes of practices pertaining to safeguard the health and safety of all workers in the workplace. They must also take precautions in their work to prevent the occurrence of any perils or infliction of injuries to themselves and their co-workers. This guide aims at introducing some relevant provisions of the Occupational Safety and Health Regulation and highlights some common hazards and their preventive measures for the workers working in elderly homes.

Manual Handling Operations

Work related to manual handling includes lifting, holding or transferring of the elders from bed to wheelchair or vice versa. Some elders who are infirm or incapable of mobility may require assistance

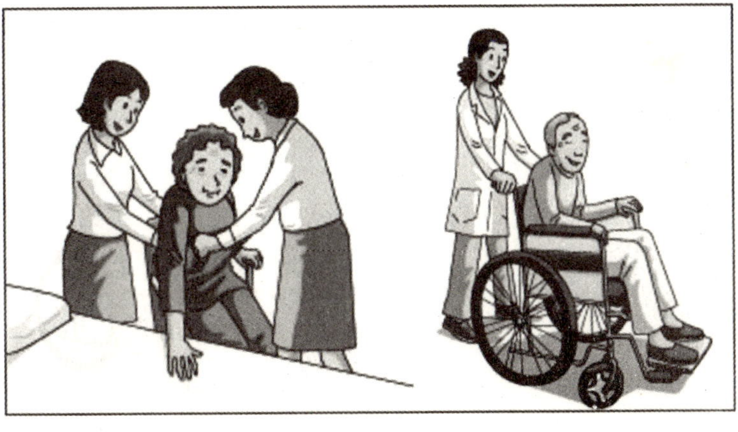

to get out of bed or change from a sitting to standing position, even in walking.

Workers who carry out lifting work with awkward posture may sustain back pain or injury. Long hours of physical demanding work with improper posture or beyond personal capability may result in musculoskeletal disorders.

Under Part VII of the Occupational Safety and Health Regulation, the employers are required to conduct a risk assessment before a manual handling operation is being undertaken by the employees. The Regulation also requires the employers to provide the preventive and protective measures for any risky manual handling operations and the necessary health and safety training for the employees.

Hints on Prevention of Injury

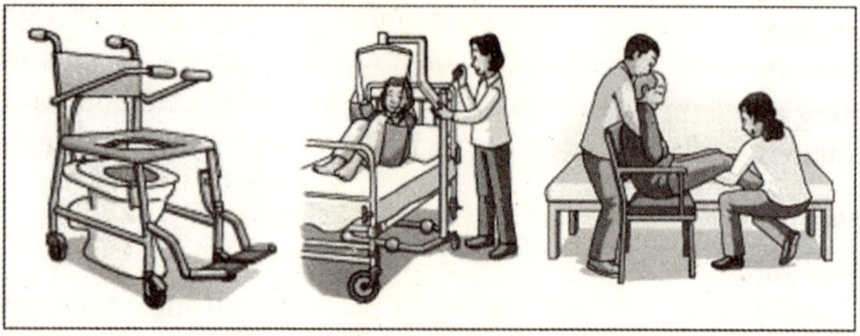

- Follow the work practices as laid down by the employers from the risk assessment findings and use mechanical aids as far as possible in lifting, holding or carrying the incapacitated elders;
- Recognize the potential risks associated with manual handling;
- Employ good posture in lifting or holding the elders and avoid excessive force, bending, twisting of the arms, wrists or neck;
- Use mechanical aids as far as possible in transporting or transferring the elders; correct operation method should be employed;
- Seek assistance from supervisor or co-workers whenever the task exceeds personal ability.

Hints on Improvement of Workplace Environment

- Maintain the work areas tidy and clean;
- Put up warning signs for wet floors immediately for any spillage of water or oil and clean-up as soon as possible;

- Use non-slippery floor materials where possible;
- Maintain the passageway and fire escape route clear of any obstruction; and
- Provide adequate lighting to the work area.

Workplace Safety

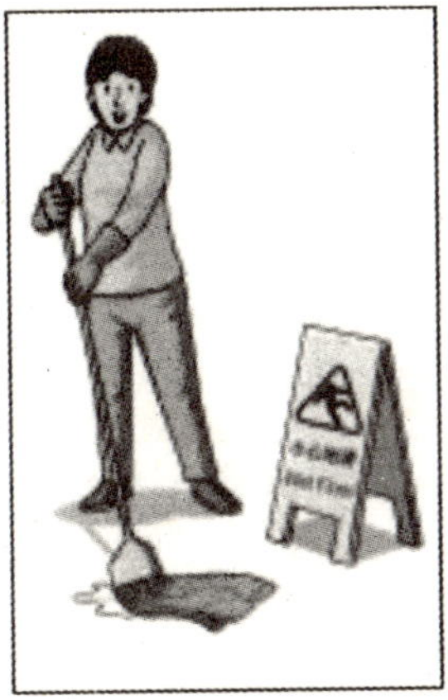

Workplace environmental conditions such as poor housekeeping, uneven or slippery floors, insufficient lighting or obstruction of the passageways and stairways are factors contributing to many accidents in the workplace. Such conditions may also lead to slips and falls as well as impede the escape in case of a fire.

Safety and Health Regulation requires the employers to ensure that the workplace environment is kept clean and adequately ventilated. The workplace must also be sufficiently well lit, by natural or artificial lighting and the floors of the workplace are adequately drained.

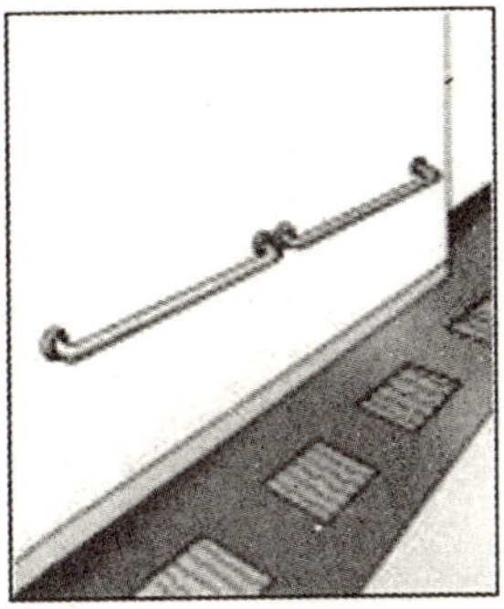

Personal Care and Nursing

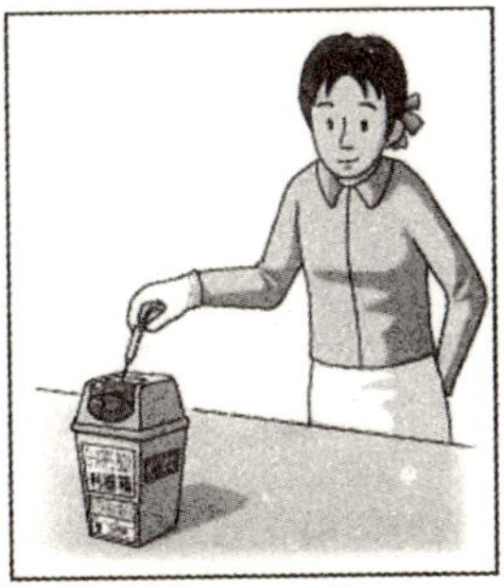

In providing personal care and nursing for the elders, the workers may use sharp instruments such as needles, scalpels and scissors which can cause injuries to them if they are not properly handled. The blood, nasal secretion, excreta, vomit and other body fluids of the infected elders may contain a large amount of bacteria and virus. Workers in contact with such materials may be infected if precautionary measures were not sufficiently taken. Under Part IV of the Occupational Safety and Health Regulation, the employers must ensure that all waste materials and debris at the workplace are kept in suitable containers. Part VI of the Regulation requires the employers to provide first aid facilities for the workers in the workplaces.

Hints on Safe Nursing

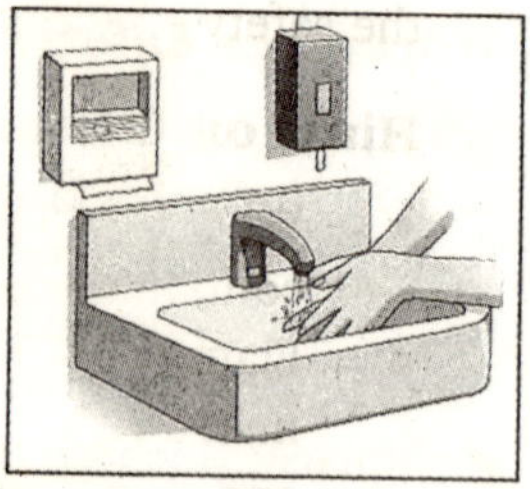

- Use needles or sharp tools with safety device; do not recap used needles;
- Discard uncapped needles with syringes and any other sharps in a labelled puncture-resistant container or sharp box for disposal;
- Provide all containers of drugs with proper labels;
- Put on gloves, masks and protective clothing in performing personal care or nursing for the elders when it is possible to come into contact with blood, body fluid or excreta;
- Pay attention to personal hygiene. Cover open areas of the skin and wounds with waterproof bandages to reduce the risk of infection;
- Wash the hands and other contaminated areas of the body thoroughly after work.

Use of Cleaning and Disinfecting Agents

Most of the commonly used cleaning agents for toilets and floors, etc., contain acidic or alkaline ingredients that may be corrosive. Some of the degreasing and stain-removing agents may contain strong organic solvents like the thinners and white spirit. These organic solvents remove the protective layer of the skin causing skin dryness or cracking leading to inflammation. Some of the organic chemicals can be absorbed into the body through the intact skin. Disinfectants including alcohol and bleaching solution may cause irritation to the skin leading to dermatitis. Corrosive chemicals in a concentrated form may cause skin burns. Incompatible chemicals when mixed can cause rigorous reactions releasing large amounts of toxic gases or fumes leading to gassing incidents. The release of toxic fumes when the beaching solution is being mixed with an acidic medium is one example. In addition, thinners, alcohols, etc., are flammable liquids. Fire and explosion may occur if they come into contact with a source of ignition or heat.

Under Part II of the Occupational Safety and Health Ordinance, the employers are required to make necessary arrangements to ensure the safety and health of employees in the use, handling, storage and transport of chemicals. Additionally, the employers are required to provide such information, instruction, training and supervision as may be necessary to ensure, so far as reasonably practicable, the safety and health at work of the employees.

Hints on Chemical Safety

- When chemicals are being used in the workplace, ensure all containers of chemicals have a proper label.
- Flammable liquid should be used clear of any heat source or naked flame; the chemicals should be kept in closed containers and stored in a strongly-constructed metal cabinet.
- Make no attempts to touch any poisonous or corrosive chemicals with bare hands. Appropriate protective gloves and safety goggles where necessary must be used when handling the chemicals.
- Volatile chemicals especially in high concentration should be used in a well ventilated work area with open windows or operating exhaust fans.
- Understand the chemical properties and pay attention to those incompatible chemicals. Never mix the incompatible chemicals and store them separately.
- In the event of any spills of the chemical on the skin, wash the affected area with a copious amount of water immediately and seek medical attention where necessary.
- In the handling of bulk chemicals, use suitable personal protective equipment such as gloves, goggles, respirators and protective clothing.
- Hands should be thoroughly washed with soap and water after handling of chemicals.
- If you have any complaints about unsafe workplaces and practices, please call the Labour Department's occupational safety and health complaint cell.

References

Gitlin, L. "Testing Home Modification Interventions: Issues of Theory, Measurement, Design and Implementation". *Annual Review of Gerontology and Geriatrics*. 18:190–237, 1998.

Pynoos, J., Tabbarah, M., Angelli, J. and Demiere, M. "Improving the Delivery of Home modification". *Technology and Disability* 8: 2–14, 1998. Published by the Occupational Safety and Health Branch of the Labour Department. Printed by the Government Logistics Department.

Ranzijn, R (2002). "The Potential of Older Adults to Enhance Community Quality of Life: Links Between Positive Psychology and Productive Ageing", Vol. 27, No 2, pp. 30–35, *Ageing Internationa.*

Sawhney, Maneeta. The Non-Governmental Organization's Commitment to the Elderly in India, Institute of Economic Growth, University Enclave, Delhi–110 007.

Stevens, M., Holman, C. D., and Bennett, N. (2001). "Preventing falls in older people: Impact of an intervention to reduce environmental hazards in the home". *Journal of the American Geriatrics Society, 49*(11), 1442–1447.

Strumpf, N., Evans, L., and Bourbonniere, M. (2001). "Restraints". In M. Mezey (ed.), *The Encyclopedia of Elder Care* (pp. 567–569). New York: Springer.

http://designforall.in/newsletter_nov_2007.pdf

http://www.workingcaregiver.com/articles/safetytips/homesafetytips

Index

age-accelerating foods, 228
age-defying foods, 227–28
ageing workforce
- in Canada, 73
- in Germany, 73–76, intervention strategies to deal with, 76
- in the EU, 73
- in the UK, 73
- in the US, 73

ageing, 3, 45, 67, 82, 157, 163, 189
- activity theory of, 214, 220
- and demographic transition, 158
- concept of, 3–4, 157–58
- in India, 4–5, 160
- process of, 3, 15, 82, 157, 170, 189–90
- role of foods in preventing, 223–24
- types of, 3, biological, 3; psychological, 3; socio-cultural, 3

Ahuja, M., M.S. Dhillon and M.S. Sandhu, 175
artificial respiration, 29–30
Avery, D.R., P.F. Mckay and D.C. Wilson, 73

Bagga, Amrita, 212, 213, 216, 217
Bhatia, H.S., 3
biological ageing, 3, 158
Blair, S.N. and S. Brodney, 150
bleeding
- first aid tips for elderly during, 32–34

Bond, John and Peter Coleman, 231
Bond, John et al., 82
Bondevik M. and A. Skogstad, 213, 214, 217, 219
Borsch-Supan, A., 75
Bose, A. and Shankardass, S., 15
breathing
- process of, 27

Casperson, C.J. et al., 150
Chadha, N.K. and P. Kanwar, 212, 213, 216, 217
Chakraborty, R.D., 163, 164, 165
Chauhan, Komal, 22
chronological ageing, 158

clothing comfort, 257
types of, 257, physical, 257; psychological, 257; social, 257
clothing, 9, 83
importance of, 44
needs for, 9–11, for elderly people, 11, 45; for elderly women, 84

D'Souza, Victor, 211, 212
Dandekar, Kumudini, 212, 215
Das, N.P. and U. Shah, 231
demographic transition, 158, 231
in India, 159
desolation, 213
Dixon, S., 73
Durnin, J.V.G.A., 150

elderly rights
in India, 169
elderly, 1, 3
dietry guidelines for, 226
in India, population of, 4–5, 15, 67, 159–61, 231, 241; rights of, 169; welfare programmes for, 169
leisure activities among, 64
malnutrition among, 16–17, factors responsible for, 16, 18
psychological problems of, 191–97
status of, in Indian society, 1, 67, 82, 83, 161–63, 171, 190, 211; initiatives to improve the, 5–8
toilet chair for, 59–60
elderly/aged women
clothing interests among, 90–143, changes in, 47–54; factors influencing, 143–44
in the world, 83
in India, status of, 174–76; role of, 176–81
emotional solitude, 213–14
extension education, 187

family, 172
Fennell, G., C. Phillipson and H. Evers, 214
fieldwork, 187
Frerichs, F. and M. Sporket, 76
functional foods, 223–24

Gangrade, K.D., 1, 2, 212
gender ageing, 83
generation gap, 2
global ageing
issue of, 73
Gopalan, C., 148
Gowli, R. Geetha, P.J. Reddy and D. Usha Rani, 82
Goyal, N., 84
graceful ageing, 166
grey population
in India, 4–5, 15, problems of, 163–66

Handler, P., 4
healthy ageing, 166
Heikkinen et al., 56
Hiebert, Paul, 219
Horwath, C.C., 18
human life
stages in, 1
Hurlock, E.B., 84

Illmarinen, J., 75
Indian society, 1, 211
changes in, 2, 82, 190, 192, 212

elderly's position in, 1, 67, 190, 192, 211–12
Irudya Rajan, S., U.S. Mishra and P.S. Sarma, 212, 213, 216

joint family system, 1–2
in India, changes in, 2, 171

Kanungo, M.N., 154
Kapadia, K.M., 219
Kaur, S. and M. Kaur, 172
Khan, I.H., 212
Kinsella, E. and V.A. Velkoff, 207
Kirpal, S. and A. Kuhl, 73, 75, 80
kiss of life (mouth-to-mouth respiration), 28–29

late middle age, 147
leisure/recreational activities, 64
importance of, 64–65, social, 66–67; economic, 67, outcomes of, 65, social, 65; creative, 65; physical, 65; emotional, 66; intellectual, 66
types of, 69–70
Limaye, Anuradha, 22

Mehta, Pallavi et al., 24
Mehta, Pallavi, Komal Chauhan and Chayanika Devi, 20
Mehta, Pallavi, Komal Chauhan and Swati Parnami, 21
Mehta, Pallavi, Monish Vyas and Mini Sheth, 17, 20
mental mendicancy, 219–20
middle age, 150
Mishra, Saraswati, 212, 216
Misra, A. and L. Khurana, 150
Morley, J.E., 16

Nalini, B., 212, 216
Nambiar, V.S. and P. Guin, 153
Nambiar, V.S. and S. Seshadri, 148, 151, 152, 154
National Policy on Older Persons (NPOP), 5, 168
nutrition transition, 147
nutrition, 223

old age diseases, 16, 30, 68
symptoms and treatment of, 30–39
old age homes, 192
comfortable living in, 242, measures for, 242–63
in India, 193–94, 212, 241–42
need for, 192–93
old age, 1, 45, 189, 231
and solitude, relations between, 214, 215–20
clothing during, 11–13, 45
health problems in, 15–17, 163–65, strategies to combat, 19–21
in Indian culture, 232
phenomenon of, 2
physiological changes during, 16, 18, 45
process of, 1
Olivares, M. et al., 19

Pan, X.R. et al., 150
Panchal, Nirali, Komal Chauhan and Pallavi Mehta, 23
parent-child relationship
in India, 192
Parthasarathy, N.R., 172
Patil, Gauri, 24
Popkin, B.M., 149
psychological ageing, 3

Ray, Sheetal, Pallavi Mehta and Komal Chauhan, 20
recreation, 63
  characteristics of, 63–64
  importance of, 64–65
  types of, 64
recreational needs
  for elderly, 67, institutional network for, 68–69
Remery, C. et al., 75, 76
role flexibility, 214
Russell, D. et al., 213

Shringarpure, Bhagyashree, 20
Singh, Dalip, 212
social isolation, 213
social solitude, 214
socio-cultural ageing, 3
solitude
  concept of, 213
  in old age, 214, 215–220
Solomons, N.W. and A.S. Anderson, 149
Soodan, K.S., 2
Sterb, C.K., S.C. Voelpel and M. Leibold, 80
successful ageing, 214
Swanson and Clarr, 187

third age, 231, 232
  time-use pattern of women in, 236–40
Tibittis, 4
toilet chair
  for elderly people, 59–60
Tucker, K.L. and S. Burnanapin, 149

unconsciousness, 34
  causes of, 34
  treatment for, 35–36

Vatuk, Sylvia, 212

women's status
  in the developing world, 83